Guides to Clinical
Aspiration Biopsy

Prostate

Guides to Clinical Aspiration Biopsy
Prostate

Tilde S. Kline, M.D.

Associate Pathologist
Chief, Division of Cytology
Lankenau Hospital

Professor of Pathology
Thomas Jefferson Medical School

Visiting Professor
Medical College of Pennsylvania
Philadelphia, Pennsylvania

IGAKU-SHOIN   New York   •   Tokyo

Interior Design by Lila G. Maron
Typesetting by Maryland Composition Company, Inc. in Garamond
Printing and Binding by Braun-Brumfield, Inc.
Cover Design by Paul Agule Design

Published and distributed by

IGAKU-SHOIN Ltd.,
5-24-3 Hongo, Bunkyo-ku, Tokyo

IGAKU-SHOIN Medical Publishers, Inc.,
1140 Avenue of the Americas, New York, N.Y. 10036

Library of Congress Cataloging in Publication Data

Kline, Tilde S., 1931–
    Prostate.

    (Guides to clinical aspiration biopsy)
    Includes bibliographies and index.
    1. Prostate gland—Cancer Diagnosis. 2. Prostate
gland—Biopsy, Needle.   3. Diagnosis, Cytologic.
4. Prostate gland—Diseases—Diagnosis.   I. Title.
[DNLM: 1. Biopsy, Needle. 2. Prostatic Diseases—
pathology.   WJ 752 K65p]
RC280.P7K55   1984   616.99'46307582   84-12957

ISBN: 0-89640-106-5 (New York)
ISBN: 4-260-14106-6 (Tokyo)

Printed and bound in U.S.A.

10 9 8 7 6 5 4 3 2 1

With gratitude to the keeper of the archives,
my associate, Ilona R. Ring

Preface

This monograph introduces the *Guides to Clinical Aspiration Biopsy*. The series is possible only because of the pioneers of the past half-century, the trio from New York's Memorial Hospital—the clinician Martin, technologist Ellis, and pathologist Stewart—who methodized this technique, and Drs. Cardozo of Holland and Söderstrom and Zajicek from Sweden, who disseminated it. Although early work was done in the United States, general interest here was dormant until the last decade. Stimulated by the rising costs of hospitalization and, currently, by the new federal regulations (e.g., Diagnostic Related Groups), aspiration biopsy has assumed its rightful place in the diagnostic regimen of the clinician and the pathologist.

At Lankenau Hospital, for more than 12 years we have applied needle aspiration biopsy (NAB) to the prostate gland and studied the aspiration biopsy cytology (ABC) of this organ by the "team approach." The urologist, skilled in patient evaluation by clinical findings, performs the NAB, customarily at the initial office examination, while the pathologist, skilled in cellular interpretation, examines the ABC; thus, two areas of expertise are combined to achieve the highest diagnostic accuracy. Needle aspiration biopsy is a highly sensitive tool, not only for clinically obvious carcinoma but also, and especially for, the equivocal lesion—the grey zone in the examination of the prostate. This monograph is based on the team approach with sections contributed by two urologists, David M. Kelsey and F. Peter Kohler. Clinical expertise was also supplied by urologists John T. Sommer and Robert B. Swain.

Aspiration biopsy cytology is presented here as a reflection of the accompanying pathology. The ABC generally is depicted in the manner the pathologist views the cells, first with the scanning lens, and finally under high magnification. Tables emphasize the salient features of the lesions. Because of the opportunity to examine tissue by a cellular approach, certain lesions, hitherto neglected, are exposed to the scrutiny of the pathologist and clinician. An example is dysplasia of the prostate, an entity in which studies are only in their infancy. In this monograph, the pathology and ABC of this fascinating lesion are presented with a review of the literature.

One of the rapidly expanding horizons in pathology is the field of immunocytochemistry. A chapter of the present volume, authored by Albert A. Keshgegian, is devoted to this subject and its application to ABC.

I would like to express my thanks to all the cytotechnologists at Lankenau Hospital who have contributed greatly to the establishment of diagnostic criteria of ABC, including Mary Ann Brown, supervisor; Mary Cahalan, Claire Sims, Lori Malloy, and Suzanne Kent. My special thanks to our Lankenau librarian, Marie Norton, for her exceptional cooperation. I am especially grateful to Michelle Darby, my dedicated secretary, and to Carol Lachowitz, cytotechnologist, for her comprehensive editing. I also would like to acknowledge the assistance of Dr. Vaidehi Kannan, cytopathologist, for meticulous measurements and observations, Dr. Betty Marchant for her tireless work in preparing the artwork for the plates, and Robert Neri for his technical aid. Special thanks are due to my photographic technologists, Tess Jennifer Kline, and her assistant, Stephan Otto Kline. I am particularly indebted to Dr. Irwin K. Kline, chief of the Department of Pathology, and to my co-pathologists, Ilona R. Ring and Joseph H. Cooper for their aid and understanding.

Tilde S. Kline, M.D.

Clinical Prologue
David M. Kelsey, M.D.

The clinical diagnosis of carcinoma of the prostate can be perturbing. Confirmation of carcinoma depends on identification of the patient with a high risk of disease and appropriate tissue sampling. Characteristically, localized cancer is asymptomatic, and, therefore, reliance on symptoms to initiate evaluation of the prostate is not satisfactory.

Since carcinoma develops in the periphery of the prostate, any associated change in consistency or configuration of the gland would be expected to be evident on transrectal examination. Indeed, the routine rectal examination is an efficient way, initially, to identify patients with high risk of prostatic malignancy.[2] There are problems, however, in accurately assessing these patients for degree of risk by palpable changes alone. Many benign-feeling glands actually harbor malignant neoplasms. Conversely, Jewett[3] reported that only 50% of his patients with a palpable, localized abnormality of the prostate, sufficiently marked and persistent to warrant open perineal biopsy, had carcinoma confirmed by histologic examination of the removed tissue. Forty percent of Colby's patients had no carcinoma following total prostatectomy not preceded by a biopsy.[1] These deficiencies persist in series done with the new forms of needle biopsy.

Ultrasound and computerized tomography can identify alteration in the configuration of the prostate, but neither technique is helpful as a screening procedure. Examination of prostatic secretions or serum studies remain questionable in evaluating the need for biopsy. Study of exfoliated cells obtained by means of prostatic massage has proved of little importance.[2,4] Thus, the confirmation of carcinoma of the prostate depends on tissue sampling.

Historically, diagnosis of carcinoma has been made by surgically obtained tissue examination. Perineal biopsy probably is the most accurate, but it requires an open operation which carries the risk of impotence. Digital-guided core-biopsy needle, either by transrectal or transperineal approach, has potential complications, and up to 25% of the biopsies may yield false-negative results. Although transurethral resection will discover or confirm an extensive carcinoma, a small, localized peripheral lesion easily can be missed.

Years ago, I was introduced to the concept of needle aspiration biopsy of the prostate.[5,6] Although I was very skeptical at first, I have come to embrace it as a superb technique. Although I always had performed a histologic-type biopsy on a stony-hard nodule, I also frequently elected surgery for the prostate with an altered consistency or symmetry or one producing rapidly changing symptoms. My concern with the formal biopsy procedure was the low but definite risk of massive bleeding, sepsis, and, rarely, death. Now, NAB may preclude the performance of a core-tissue needle biopsy.

The technique of NAB is straightforward and can be learned in a brief time. The equipment is readily available in any hospital or office. I have never found it necessary to use the special fine-needle finger-guide and syringe-gun developed and suggested in Sweden. The patient requires no special instructions and no enemas. The prostate is palpated in the ordinary manner. With the index finger of one hand, the 18- to 22-gauge spinal needle is directed to the suspicious area and then attached to a disposable 10-cc syringe; there it is advanced and withdrawn slightly several times, as negative pressure is applied through the syringe. The needle then is removed, and the sample is ejected onto previously prepared, albuminized slides and thinly smeared and fixed. Several specimens are obtained. The slides may be preserved indefinitely in alcohol until they are processed.

In our series, correlation of the aspiration biopsy and core-needle biopsy has been over 90% accurate.[7] The results can be available within 1 hour. Thus, we can avoid causing the patient excessive anxiety, and yet we can counsel him before the significance of the problem is lost.

How safe is the procedure? From more than 1,500 patients we have had four complications; three patients developed fever requiring treatment and one was briefly hospitalized because of his poor general physical condition. At no time have we seen any bleeding.

I find NAB of great value in patients with somewhat firm glands (e.g., after transurethral resection), in patients with recent change in voiding pattern, for follow-up after radiation therapy to the prostate, and in patients with possible prostatitis in whom a core biopsy could be especially dangerous. A negative ABC, in such circumstances, is a meaningful diagnostic result. On the other hand, if the gland is very suspicious, a negative result is meaningless. Following a suspicious report, I repeat the NAB as frequently as necessary or perform a core biopsy.

I still tend to confirm the positive ABC with core biopsy. However, my associates do not feel that this usually is mandatory, particularly in moderately to poorly differentiated carcinomas. I also do not confirm the positive aspirate from the elderly, debilitated patient for whom there is a potentially severe risk with core biopsy. Another advantage of a positive ABC is that it gives additional encouragement to any other necessary type of biopsy. It allows rapid and sensible planning of indicated tests. Bone scan and admission can be arranged, and the patient can be informed of the length of hospitalization and possible need for either radical or palliative surgery.

The following two cases demonstrate the value of aspiration biopsy:

> A 63-year-old man was referred because of an enlarged prostate with a nodule of the right lobe. Both core biopsy and aspiration biopsy were done with conflicting results. Core biopsy revealed focal dysplasia (see Chapter 9), and ABC was suggestive of well-differentiated

carcinoma. Since repeat NAB revealed well-differentiated carcinoma, an open perineal biopsy was done, and the carcinoma was confirmed.

A 71-year-old man presented with decreased stream. On physical examination, a right-sided prostatic nodule was found. Needle aspiration biopsy revealed cells consistent with moderately differentiated carcinoma, but the core biopsy revealed only benign disease. On evaluation, however, intravenous pyelogram delineated a left renal mass which proved to be a hypernephroid carcinoma. Six months later with the prostate almost normal on palpation, NAB was again repeated and again was reported as possible carcinoma, but a repeat core biopsy was benign. When a third ABC was reported as positive, I performed an open perineal biopsy. This showed a moderately differentiated adenocarcinoma, and I treated his second carcinoma appropriately.

Without aspiration biopsy in both of these cases, the carcinoma would have been missed entirely (see Figs. 9.1 and 9.2).

Here is a reliable method which is easy to master. Any suspicious area can be safely and rapidly investigated in the office as part of a routinely scheduled appointment. Needle aspiration biopsy is a guide to the patient and the physician, and it fulfills the need for an efficient means to screen suspicious glands.

REFERENCES

1. Colby FH: Carcinoma of the prostate; results of total prostatectomy. *J Urol* 69:797–806, 1963.

2. Guinan P, Bush I, Ray V, Vieth R, Rao R, Bhatti R: The accuracy of the rectal examination in the diagnosis of prostatic carcinoma. *N Engl J Med* 303:499–503, 1980.

3. Jewett HJ: Significance of the palpable prostatic nodule. *JAMA* 160:838–839, 1956.

4. Kaufman JJ, Rosenthal M, Goodwin WE: Methods of diagnosis of carcinoma of the prostate: a comparison of clinical impression, prostatic smear, needle biopsy, open perineal biopsy and transurethral biopsy. *J Urol* 72:450–463, 1954.

5. Kelsey DM, Kohler FP, MacKinney CC, Kline TS: Out-patient needle aspiration biopsy of the prostate. *J Urol* 116:327–328, 1976.

6. Kline TS, Kelsey DM, Kohler FP: Prostatic carcinoma and needle aspiration biopsy. *Am J. Clin Pathol* 67:131–133, 1977.

7. Kline TS, Kohler FP, Kelsey DM: Aspiration biopsy cytology (ABC); its use in diagnosis of lesions of the prostate gland. *Arch Pathol Lab Med* 106:136–139, 1982.

Contributors

David M. Kelsey, M.D.
Associate, Divison of Urology
Department of Surgery
Lankenau Hospital
and
Clinical Associate Professor of Urology
Thomas Jefferson University School of Medicine
Philadelphia, Pennsylvania

Albert A. Keshgegian, M.D., Ph.D.
Associate Pathologist
Lankenau Hospital
and
Adjunct Assistant Professor, Pathology and
   Laboratory Medicine
University of Pennsylvania School of Medicine
Philadelphia, Pennsylvania

F. Peter Kohler, M.D.
Chief, Division of Urology
Lankenau Hospital
and
Associate Professor of Urology
Thomas Jefferson University School of Medicine
Philadelphia, Pennsylvania

Contents

KEY TO ABBREVIATIONS

ABC   Aspiration Biopsy Cytology

NAB   Needle Aspiration Biopsy

1

Introduction

Carcinoma of the prostate is the second most common malignant neoplasm in men. It affects 18% of the male population, causes almost 10% of all cancer deaths, and current, newly discovered cases will number approximately 75,000.[37] From a study of 4,696 consecutive autopsies, there were 412 (9%) prostatic carcinomas, 188 diffuse and 224 focal.[21] The incidence rises with age and ranges from 26 to 52% in men over the age of 80 years.[21,22]

Prostatic carcinoma has its counterpart in carcinoma of the cervix, but unlike the latter, which often is discovered by exfoliative cytology, it seldom is detected early. Carcinoma, when confined to the prostate (stages A and B) and treatable by a variety of methods, is usually symptom-free. Flocks,[18] investigating 4,000 patients with carcinoma, reported that only 10% were discovered during routine physical examination, whereas 80% already had symptoms of lower urinary tract obstruction at the time of diagnosis.

Many methods for tissue sampling of the prostate are available, but the majority require hospitalization, special patient preparation, and anesthesia, and may cause significant complications. The most accurate is open perineal biopsy since it exposes the entire outer area of the prostate; yet, it necessitates general anesthesia, and it may result in impotence. Core-needle biopsy through the perineum or rectum selectively samples the outer zone and requires only local anesthesia. The complication rate, however, is 13–51%; complications include not only fever, hematuria, and cystitis, but occasionally fistulae, sepsis[4,6,8] and, rarely, death.[43] There also have been a few accounts of tumor seeding along the needle tract.[5,9,34] Least accurate for detection of stage A and B carcinoma is transurethral resection, primarily from the central zone. In a comparative study of open perineal biopsy, core biopsy and transurethral resection, Kaufman et al[24] detected 10% of 27 stage A carcinomas by core-needle biopsy and the remainder only by open perineal biopsy; in patients with advanced disease, 40% were verified by transurethral resection and 76% by core biopsy.

Prior to most forms of biopsy, the index of suspicion must be high, whereas NAB can be used for a mildly suspicious area. Thus, Mostofi, dean of urologic pathologists, has remarked that this technique may shortly supplant core biopsy.[31] It is anticipated that NAB will become increasingly important for early diagnosis, and possibly for screening programs for men over age 50. In an editorial on current concepts of prostatic carcinoma, Olsson[32] commented: "It is becoming increasingly clear that this technique [aspiration biopsy] will necessarily become a part of the practicing urologist's diagnostic armamentarium. . . . The medical and economic advantages need no additional comment. . . . Furthermore . . . a simple screening test for adenocarcinoma of the prostate is needed."

HISTORY

In 1930, Russell Ferguson, a urologist from New York's Memorial Hospital, published his report, "Prostatic neoplasms: their diagnosis by needle puncture and aspiration."[17] Crediting Martin and Ellis from his institution, Ferguson applied the technique to the prostate by traversing the perineum with an 18-gauge needle attached to a Record syringe and successfully procured prostatic cells in first 70%, and later in 86% of his patients.[16] Emphasizing the importance of an "able and willing" pathologist, he pointed out the usefulness of the procedure for detecting primary prostatic carcinoma in two patients with occult metastatic carcinoma to the lung. The "able and willing" pathologist, Stewart, upon interpretation of 194 aspirates, described the malignant cells as "usually diffusely arranged and distinct alveolar characteristics are lacking. They are larger, disconnected and more atypical than the cells of benign hyperplasia."[40]

Scant attention was paid to these innovative studies for two decades. Urologists developed skill in use of the 2.0- to 3.5-mm core biopsy tools rather than the 0.6 to 0.9-mm fine needles. Needle aspiration biopsy was adopted in Sweden's Karolinska Institute in 1956 and modified by Franzén[19] who approached the prostate through the rectum. He adapted a curved needle with a finger-guide which he attached to a syringe gun and reported on 100 transrectal aspiration biopsies, a study implemented by Esposti with 1,110 patients.[13] In 1969, Rheinfrank and Nulf,[35] using the new approach, reintroduced the method in the United States with a report of 209 aspirates, including 23 carcinomas, and described it as "an office procedure for routine screening for carcinoma of the prostate." By 1976, multinational reporters included Bachmann[3] from Switzerland, Williams et al[44] from England, Alfthan et al[2] from Finland, Sparwasser and Lüchtrath[38] from Germany, Pellet and Gretillat[33] from France, Cardozo[7] from Holland, Epstein[11] from South Africa, and also, from Germany, Staehler et al[39] who produced a color atlas.

At Lankenau Hospital in 1974, we began our studies as an adjunct to core-needle biopsy and as an ancillary office procedure.[25,26,28] All specimens were taken by the urologists with disposable equipment, a thin-gauge spinal needle without a finger guide and a syringe without a syringe-holder. Currently, we examine approximately 300 patients a year, of which 30% have carcinoma. The results, dealing with examination of our more than 1500 patients, and a review of the literature, are presented on the following pages.

INDICATIONS

What are the indications for fine-needle aspiration biopsy of the prostate? Von Reuter and Schuck[41] stated that because it is almost as easy as rectal palpation, it always should supplement that procedure. Esposti,[12] however, believed it only should be applied to clinically suspicious nodules since, in the immense series from Radiumhemmet, these were the glands in which carcinoma had been uncovered by the fine needle. Staehler et al[39] wrote that induration was an absolute indication for the procedure. Hendry[23] suggested NAB for the first examination and repetition when indicated, but he recommended core biopsy if the findings did not verify the initial impression. Ward[42] believed that the techniques should complement each other. The indications for NAB may be summarized:

1. All glands with altered consistency by palpation
2. All glands with inconclusive tissue biopsies
3. Indurated glands following transurethral resection
4. Staging prostatic carcinoma
5. All glands in men over age 50 with occult metastatic carcinoma
6. All glands following therapy for prostatic carcinoma

COMPLICATIONS

The complication rate of NAB from the prostate varies from 1 to 7%. There have been no reports of tumor implantation seeded by the fine needle. Esposti et al[14] from their first 3,000 NABs had 12 patients with minor complications including epididymitis, hematuria, hemospermia, and fever, an incidence of 0.4% which increased to 7.1% when they took biopsies from patients with rheumatoid disorders. Others[15,38,39,41] reported minor complications ranging in frequency from 1 to 6%. From our series, there have been a few patients with transient fever, an incidence of less than 1%.

CONTRASTS:
ASPIRATION BIOPSY CYTOLOGY
AND EXFOLIATIVE CYTOLOGY

Interpretation of ABC both resembles and differs from interpretation of exfoliative cytology. Aspiration biopsy cytology is based on pattern alterations, whereas exfoliative cytology is based on individual cell alterations. The scanning lens ($\times 2.5$) is vital for at least the initial examination of ABC, but it is used infrequently for exfoliative cytology. In our institution, neither cytopathologists nor cytotechnol-

TABLE 1.1. General Diagnostic Criteria

ABC	Benignity	Malignancy
Cellularity	+	+ + +
Cohesion	+ + +	+
Nuclear membrane regularity	+ + +	±
Anisonucleosis	−	+ +
Eosinophilic macronucleoli	−	+ +
Distinct cell borders	+ + +	±
Polarization	+ + +	±

ogists use the mechanical stage because of the importance of the preliminary and final scan for inspection of the ABC.

Diagnostic criteria for aspiration biopsy cytology deviate from those for exfoliative cytology (Table 1.1). The two most important judgmental criteria for ABC are cellularity and dyshesion (defined as "disordered cell adherence; loss of intercellular cohesion," in Dorland's Medical Dictionary, 26th ed), by contrast to hyperchromasia and pleomorphism for exfoliated cells. Important common criteria include aniso-nucleosis (variation of nuclear size), nuclear membrane irregularity and eosinophilic macronucleoli (at least 1.25 μm), while mitoses are rare in both. Nuclear/cyto-plasmic ratio alteration and a sanguineous, inflammatory diathesis, significant in exfoliative cytology, play minimal roles in diagnosis of ABC: neutrophils, necrotic debris and blood are more often associated with inflammation and abscess than with malignant tumors. All ABC criteria may not be present in a single case, but a majority of these criteria will be evident (see Chapter 7).

The aspirate from a benign lesion frequently is cell-poor. The cells form large, cohesive, uniform groups. McCutcheon et al[30] tested the ease of cell dislodgment and found marked adhesiveness in benign tissue. Cell borders are distinct, and nuclear membranes are regular (see Chapter 4).

Thus, it is apparent that a bridge must be traversed from interpretation of ex-foliative cytology to interpretation of ABC. When these special diagnostic criteria are recognized and each specimen is screened for them, ABC usually is swiftly and accurately interpreted.

DIAGNOSTIC PHRASEOLOGY

In our laboratory, diagnosis by ABC is reported similarly to histologic diagnosis. For benign diagnoses, a meaningful statement is employed in place of "negative" ("denoting the absence of something," *Webster's College Dictionary*, 1977):

Cells compatible with benign prostatic enlargement.

Cells compatible with chronic prostatitis.

No malignant tumor cells seen. Rather scant aspirate.

A report of "unsatisfactory" establishes the specific cause. Factors include insufficient numbers of cells from the prostate, poor cell preservation, blood which obscures underlying cells, and seminal vesicle contamination (see Chapter 9, section on Interpretative Traps).

Sometimes a "suspicious" report must be issued. It is used when the cells display insufficient diagnostic criteria of malignancy, or when there are findings which may cause diagnostic pitfalls (see Chapter 9). Terminology includes:

Atypia, perhaps secondary to prostatitis.

Marked cellularity with a few atypical cells.

Atypia, perhaps secondary to seminal vesicle contamination.

A few cells suggestive of well-differentiated adenocarcinoma.

In our institution, in addition to a written evaluation, we also discuss the case with the clinician who may repeat the aspirate, treat for infection, or take a core biopsy. A number of these patients, after long-term follow-up, have had proven carcinomas (see Chapter 9).

Aspirates are designated as "positive for carcinoma" when the criteria of malignancy are met. Whenever possible, the malignant cells also are classified according to the degree of differentiation (see Chapter 6). Occasionally, we suggest the possibility of a primary carcinoma arising outside the prostate (see Chapter 6, section on Secondary Malignancies).

STATISTICS

Accuracy of fine-needle aspiration biopsy is difficult to gauge because of inherent difficulties in obtaining adequate tissue samples from the prostate (see Chapter 9). The predictive value of positive results ranges from 68 to 91% in studies with at least 50 tissue-confirmed carcinomas. [Sensitivity = (TP/TP + FN) × 100%; specificity = (TN/TN + FP) × 100%; F, false; N, negative; P, positive; T, true; suspicious diagnoses are excluded from calculation.][20] It is noteworthy that the accuracy of the technique is independent of the use of specially designed equipment (Table 1.2).

TABLE 1.2. Biopsy-Verified Carcinomas

Author	Cases of Carcinoma	Franzén Needle	ABC Sensitivity
Ackermann[1]	229	Yes	82%
Alfthan[2]	82	?	84%
Esposti[13]	58	Yes	91%
Kline[27]	158	No	85%
Lin[29]	203	Yes	68%
Schulte-Wissermann[36]	130	No	87%
VonReuter[41]	54	No	75%

TABLE 1.3. Unsatisfactory Reports

Author	Total No. Cases	Franzén Needle	Unsat. ABC
Ackermann[1]	645	Yes	6.4%
Epstein[11]	118	No	2.5%
Esposti[13]	1,110	Yes	2 %
Faul[15]	350	Yes	7.1%
Hendry[23]	138	Yes	10 %
Kline[27]	540	No	2.6%
Lin[29]	1,280	Yes	6 %

From our study of 540 lesions with 158 proven carcinomas and 158 biopsy-verified benign lesions,[27] sensitivity was 85% and specificity 91%. The sensitivity rose upon application of minor criteria of malignancy for diagnosis of well-differentiated carcinoma (see Chapter 6). Others have reported that a subsequent second or even third NAB enhances the sensitivity.[46] The specificity, too, undoubtably is greater because of the carcinomas which are unconfirmed due to inadequacy of tissue biopsy techniques. We and others[10,11,13,15,27,29] have established that by repeated tissue biopsy, the ABC "false-positive" result usually becomes the "true-positive" (see Chapter 9).

In series with more than 100 patients, unsatisfactory specimens range from 2 to 10% (Table 1.3). These figures demonstrate that an adequate aspirate is unrelated to the biopsy tools. Groups using the Franzén needle and syringe-gun provide neither higher sensitivity nor fewer unsatisfactory specimens than those using the simple "spinal" needle and disposable syringe. The single exception occurs in the Karolinska Institute, where the Franzén needle was developed, after 20 years experience on more than 15,000 patients. Three physicians perform all biopsies on 750 patients yearly with an unsatisfactory rate of only 0.7%.[12,45]

REFERENCES

1. Ackermann R, Müller HA: Retrospective analysis of 645 simultaneous perineal punch biopsies and transrectal aspiration biopsies for diagnosis of prostatic carcinoma. *Eur Urol* 3:29–34, 1977.

2. Alfthan O, Klintrup HE, Koivuniemi A, Taskinen E: Cytological aspiration biopsy and Vim-Silverman biopsy in the diagnosis of prostatic carcinoma. *Ann Chir Gynaecol Fenn* 59:226–229, 1970.

3. Bachmann KF: Cytodiagnostische untersuchung der Prostata mit transrectaler Aspirations-punktion. *Schweiz Med Wochenschr* 96:1225–1227, 1966.

4. Bartelsen S: Transrectal needle biopsy of the prostate. *Acta Chir Scand,* suppl. 357:226–231, 1966.

5. Blackard CE, Soucheray JA, Gleason DF: Prostatic needle biopsy with perineal extension of adenocarcinoma. *J Urol* 106:401–403, 1971.

6. Brawn PN: *Interpretation of Prostate Biopsies*. New York, Raven Press, 1983.

7. Cardozo PL: *Atlas Clinical Cytology*. The Netherlands, Targa b.v.'s-Hertogenbosch, 1975, pp. 527–537.

8. Davison P, Malament M: Urinary contamination as a result of transrectal biopsy of the prostate. *J Urol* 105:545–546, 1971.

9. Desai SLG, Woodruff LM: Carcinoma of prostate; local extension following perineal needle biopsy. *Urology* 3:87–88, 1974.

10. Ekman H, Hedberg K, Persson PS: Cytological versus histological examination of needle biopsy specimens in the diagnosis of prostatic cancer. *Br J Urol* 39:544–548, 1967.

11. Epstein NA: Prostatic biopsy; a morphologic correlation of aspiration cytology with needle biopsy histology. *Cancer* 38:2078–2087, 1976.

12. Esposti PL: Aspiration biopsy and cytologic evaluation for primary diagnosis and follow-up. In Jacob, GH, Hohenfellner R: *Prostate Cancer. International Prospectives in Urology*, vol 3. Baltimore, Williams and Wilkins, 1982, pp. 71–92.

13. Esposti PL: Cytologic diagnosis of prostatic tumors with the aid of transrectal aspiration biopsy; a critical review of 1110 cases and a report of morphologic and cytochemical studies. *Acta Cytol* 10:182–186, 1966.

14. Esposti PL, Elman A, Norlen H: Complications of transrectal aspiration biopsy of the prostate. *Scand J Urol Nephrol* 9:208–213, 1975.

15. Faul P, Schmiedt E: Cytologic aspects of diseases of the prostate. *Int Urol Nephrol* 5:297–310, 1973.

16. Ferguson RS: Diagnosis and treatment of early carcinoma of the prostate. *J Urol* 37:774–782, 1937.

17. Ferguson RS: Prostatic neoplasms: their diagnosis by needle puncture and aspiration. *Am J Surg* 9:507–511, 1930.

18. Flocks RH: Clinical cancer of the prostate; a study of 4000 cases. *JAMA* 193:559–562, 1965.

19. Franzén S, Giertz G, Zajicek J: Cytological diagnosis of prostatic tumours by transrectal aspiration biopsy: a preliminary report. *Br J Urol* 32:193–196, 1960.

20. Galen RS, Gambino SR: *Beyond Normality: The Predictive Value and Efficiency of Medical Diagnosis*. New York, John Wiley & Sons, 1975.

21. Halpert B, Sheehan EE, Schmalhorst WR, Scott R: Carcinoma of the prostate; a survey of 5000 autopsies. *Cancer* 16:737–742, 1963.

22. Harbitz TB, Haugen OA: Histology of the prostate in elderly men; a study in an autopsy series. *Acta Pathol Microbiol Scand* 80:756–768, 1972.

23. Hendry WF, Williams JP: Transrectal prostatic biopsy. *Br Med J* 4:595–597, 1971.

24. Kaufman JJ, Rosenthal M, Goodwin WE: Methods of diagnosis of carcinoma of the prostate: a comparison of clinical impression, prostatic smear, needle biopsy, open perineal biopsy and transurethral biopsy. *J Urol* 72:450–463, 1954.

25. Kelsey DM, Kohler FP, MacKinney CC, Kline TS: Out-patient needle aspiration biopsy of the prostate. *J Urol* 116:327–328, 1976.

26. Kline TS, Kelsey DM, Kohler FP: Prostatic carcinoma and needle aspiration biopsy. *Am J Clin Pathol* 67:131–133, 1977.

27. Kline TS, Kohler FP, Kelsey DM: Aspiration biopsy cytology (ABC); its use in diagnosis of lesions of the prostate gland. *Arch Pathol Lab Med* 106:136–139, 1982.

28. Kohler FP, Kelsey DM, MacKinney CC, Kline TS: Needle aspiration of the prostate. *J Urol* 118:1012, 1977.

29. Lin BPC, Davies WEL, Harmata PA: Prostatic aspiration cytology. *Pathology* 11:607–617, 1979.

30. McCutcheon M, Coman DR, Moore FB: Studies on invasiveness of cancer; adhesiveness of malignant cells in various human adenocarcinomas. *Cancer* 1:460–467, 1948.

31. Mostofi FK: Progress in urologic pathology. Medical College of Pennsylvania, April 13, 1982.

32. Olsson CA: Aspiration biopsy of the prostate: editorial comment. *Semin Urol* 1:176, 1983.

33. Pellet A, Gretillat PA: Diagnostic cytologique des tumeurs prostatiques par ponction transrectale a l'aiguille fine de Franzen; revue de 90 cas. *Ann Urol* 5:247–252, 1971.

34. Puigvert A, Elizalde C, Matz JA: Perineal implantation of carcinoma of the prostate following needle biopsy: a case report. *J Urol* 107:821–824, 1972.

35. Rheinfrank RE, Nulf TH: Fine needle aspiration biopsy of the prostate. *Endoscopy* 1:27–32, 1969.

36. Schulte-Wissermann H, Lüchtrath H: Aspiration biopsie und Cytologie beim Prosta-tacarcinom. *Virchows Arch [Pathol Anat]* 352:122–129, 1971.

37. Silverberg E: Cancer statistics, 1984. *CA* 33:7–23, 1984.

38. Sparwasser H, Lüchtrath H: Die transrectale Saugbiopsie der biopsie der Prostate. *Urologe* 9:281–285, 1970.

39. Staehler W, Ziegler H, Völter D, Schubert GE: *Color Atlas of Cytodiagnosis of the Prostate*. Stuttgart, FK Schattauer Verlag, 1975.

40. Stewart FW: The diagnosis of tumors by aspiration. *Am J Pathol* 9:801–812, 1933.

41. VonReuter HJ, Schuck W: Die Nadelbiopsie der Prostata zur Zytologischen Karzinom-diagnostik Erfahrungen an 1500 Fällen. *Z Urol Nephrol* 64:857–862, 1971.

42. Ward JP: Franzen-needle transrectal prostatic biopsy. *Lancet* 2:327–328, 1973.

43. Wendel RG, Evans AT: Complications of punch biopsy of the prostate. *J Urol* 97:122–126, 1967.

44. Williams JP, Still BM, Pugh RCB: The diagnosis of prostatic cancer: cytological and biochemical studies using the Franzen biopsy needle. *Br J Urol* 39:549–554, 1967.

45. Willems JS, Löwhagen T: Transrectal fine-needle aspiration biopsy for cytologic diagnosis and grading of prostatic carcinoma. *The Prostate* 2:381–395, 1981.

46. Zajicek J: *Aspiration Biopsy Cytology. Part II. Cytology of Infradiaphragmatic Organs*. Basel, Karger, 1979, pp. 129–166.

2

Clinical and Laboratory Techniques

NEEDLE ASPIRATION BIOPSY

The Prostate

Needle aspiration biopsy (NAB) of the prostate is an office or bedside procedure. Hospitalization, prior patient preparation, and antibiotics are unnecessary. The patient stands, bent forward over the examining table, lies in the lithotomy position or, if bedridden, is positioned on his side with legs flexed. No anesthetic agent is needed. Enhanced cellularity is achieved, however, if the needle is dampened with a few drops of Xylocaine prior to biopsy. A 20- or 22-gauge, 90-mm (spinal) disposable needle with obturator, is placed against the index finger with its tip immediately proximal to the end of the finger. The index finger with its molded needle is advanced into the rectum to the site where the suspicious nodule is palpated. Finally, the needle is pushed through the rectal wall into the adjacent abnormal area of the prostate (Figs. 2.1–2.3). With the free hand, the obturator is withdrawn, a 10-cc disposable syringe is attached, and negative pressure is applied by depression of the plunger while advancing and withdrawing the needle several times in different planes. The needle is removed after release of pressure; failure to release pressure results in rectal contamination. The minute specimen usually is entirely within the needle. It is expelled forcibly onto one end of a slide without contact of the needle tip with the slide. The specimen usually consists of several viscid, yellow-white, or blood-tinged droplets comprising approximately 0.1–0.3 cc. While still moist, the droplets must be spread to a thin film and fixed immediately (see section on Specimen Preparation, below). For adequate sampling, at least two biopsies must be performed, reusing the same equipment. A large fluid sample almost always indicates urine and is unsatisfactory.

The tools for all our biopsies are the disposable 18- to 22-gauge, 90-mm spinal needle and disposable 10-cc syringe. Neither a special needle with finger-guide nor

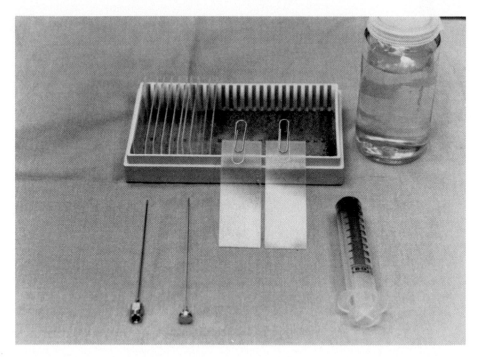

Fig. 2.1. Equipment: syringe, 20-gauge spinal needle with obturator, slides, and fixative.

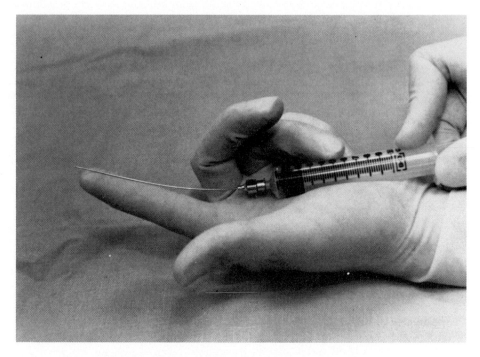

Fig. 2.2. The needle is molded to the index finger.

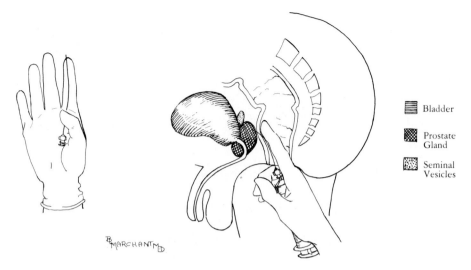

Bladder

Prostate
Gland

Seminal
Vesicles

Fig. 2.3. Needle aspiration biopsy of the prostate.

syringe-gun are needed for good specimens. Clinicians can easily master the technique, and have no problem presenting satisfactory material to the pathologist (Tables 2.1 and 2.2).

TABLE 2.1. Needle Aspiration Biopsy Technique

1. Advance needle into suspicious nodule.
2. Attach syringe and apply negative pressure.
3. Rotate needle in stabbing motions.
4. Release negative pressure and withdraw needle.
5. Eject specimen vigorously onto slide.
6. Fix immediately.
7. Repeat steps 1–6 for a total of two or three passes.

TABLE 2.2. Preparation

1. Eject specimen vigorously onto prepared slide.
2. Spread droplets to thin film, rapidly.
3. Fix immediately.
4. Stain.

Superficial Soft Tissue Masses

For examination of superficial soft tissue masses adjacent to or distant from the prostate, NAB is invaluable (see Chapter 8). Instruments for puncture are the 22-gauge, 30-mm disposable needle and 3- to 5-cc disposable Leur-Lok syringe. With the syringe attached to a 25-gauge needle, 0.5 cc Xylocaine is injected to raise a wheal at the periphery of the lesion. Thus, the Xylocaine neither obscures the mass nor dilutes the sample because of dermal infiltration. Then the 25-gauge needle is replaced by a 22-gauge needle, and the Xylocaine remaining in the syringe is flushed out through the needle, leaving it moist but fluid free. The needle, positioned within the mass, is rotated back and forth in a fan-like and/or corkscrew motion under negative pressure. After release of the plunger, the needle is withdrawn with the specimen usually confined within the needle. Three passes are advised. When the lesion is large, these should be made at the periphery since the central area may consist only of necrotic debris.

Bone

Needle aspiration biopsy is a valuable tool for osteolytic and osteoblastic bone lesions in patients with known or suspected prostatic carcinoma. For osteolytic tumors, NAB is taken with the same equipment as for superficial masses, but a 22-gauge, 90-mm (spinal) or 120-mm (Chiba) needle may be substituted in the obese patient. The needle is inserted through the skin directly into the bony site, often the point of maximal tenderness. The biopsy procedure is similar to that for soft-tissue masses, but the needle must be rotated gently to prevent hemodilution. For large osteolytic lesions this is an office procedure, whereas for small lesions, for those involving the vertebrae, or for positive areas demonstrated by bone scan, positioning of the needle is performed under fluoroscopic or computerized tomographic guidance. Radiographic guidance is also used for NAB of osteoblastic tumors. Since a fine needle cannot pierce these lesions, a trephine needle (e.g., Jamshidi or Turkel) is requisite for bone penetration. Then the 22-gauge needle is threaded through its lumen, and the customary two or three passes are made.

SPECIMEN PREPARATION

In our laboratory we routinely process slide-filmed specimens according to the method of Papanicolaou (Table 2.2) for clarity of cellular detail. Other laboratories process air-dried films with May-Grünwald Giemsa or Diff Quik stain. Yet other investigators collect specimens in fluid and process them by membrane filter or paraffin-embedded cell block techniques, but these procedures are costly and time consuming for general usage, negating two important advantages of NAB.

The specimen is ejected onto a glass slide. Prior slide-coating with albumin enhances cellular adherance before fixation by alcohol, but is unnecessary before fixation by special spray or Carbowax. A monolayered film can be made in two ways: the simpler is to smear the droplets rapidly with a second albuminized slide or applicator stick (one to two slides per pass). Alternatively, a more concentrated film can be made (Fig. 2.4). A clean slide or coverslip is touched to the ejected droplets which are caught onto its edge by a sweeping motion. This specimen-containing slide-edge is rubbed focally with a quick, light motion against a fresh slide to make the film. The first method is easier to master, whereas the second provides a consolidated aspirate, adhering without albumin, which can be screened rapidly. Note, however, that for evaluation of cellularity, a major criterion of malignancy, the first

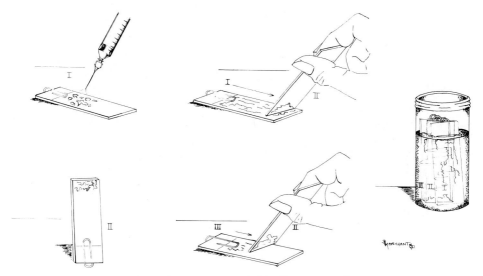

Fig. 2.4. Concentrated thin-film preparation.

method provides a lower cell density than the second (see Chapter 9, section on Interpretative Traps).

For preparation by the Papanicolaou method, fixation must be immediate while the specimen is still moist. Fixation is the same regardless of slide preparation technique and is accomplished by one of the following methods:

1. 95% alcohol (ethyl or methyl)
2. Carbowax solution (see section on Specimen Preparation, below)
3. Aerosal spray (e.g., hair spray or commercial fixative)

We prefer 95% alcohol fixative because it causes minimal cell distortion. In addition, the slides may be stained within 2 minutes of fixation without prolonged alcohol immersion for dissolution of a spray fixative. Speed is essential in our busy laboratory where the clinician often requests immediate diagnosis. When slides are to be transported from office to laboratory, we suggest Carbowax or a spray fixative which should be applied at an approximate distance of 8 in. from the slide. Otherwise the cells may be propelled to the edge of the slide or unevenly preserved. Once the fixative is applied to the specimen, the process can be interrupted indefinitely.

Carbowax

Polyethylene glycol solution
95% ethyl or methyl alcohol

1. Mix 1 part polyethylene glycol solution with 15 parts alcohol solution.
2. Place three drops on the specimen-containing slide. This coats the slide with a thin film of wax.

Papanicolaou stain is routinely applied to all slides in our laboratory.

Routine Papanicolaou Stain*

Spray or Carbowax fixative: begin with step 1
Alcohol fixative: begin with step 2

1.	95% ethyl alcohol	5–10 minutes
2.	Tap water	1 minute
3.	Hematoxylin (Gill's)	1 minute
4.	Tap water	1–2 minutes
5.	95% ethyl alcohol	1 minute
6.	Orange 6	1 minute
7.	95% ethyl alcohol	1 minute
8.	Eosin-azure 65	1 minute
9.	95% ethyl alcohol	1 minute
10.	Absolute alcohol	1 minute
11.	Xylol	2 minutes (until clear)
12.	Mount	

* *Note:* Methyl can be substituted for ethyl alcohol. Stains change strength, and the timing varies according to usage and storage conditions.

Special stains can be substituted for the Papanicolaou stain or applied following decolorization of the specimen:

Decolorization of Papanicolaou-Stained Smears*

Procedure:

1.	Remove coverslip in xylol	
2.	Absolute alcohol	2 minutes
3.	95% ethyl alcohol	1 minute
4.	Tap water	1 minute
5.	0.05% aqueous hydrochloric acid	5–30 minutes
6.	Tap water	2 minutes

* (From Sachdeva R, Kline TS: Aspiration biopsy cytology and special stains. *Acta Cytol* 25:678–683, 1981.)

Almost all histochemical stains can be applied to the ABC specimen.[1] For differentiating a mucin-producing adenocarcinoma of the rectum from a prostatic carcinoma, the mucicarmine stain is helpful:

Mucicarmine Stain*

Components:

1. Mayers mucicarmine solution (Polyscientific Laboratory): mix one part with four parts tap water prior to use
2. Hematoxylin

Procedure (35–40 minutes):

1.	Counterstain nuclei in hematoxylin.	1–5 minutes
2.	Tap water	$\frac{1}{2}$ minute
3.	Stain in Mayers Mucicarmine solution.	30 minutes
4.	Tap water	$\frac{1}{2}$ minute
5.	Dehydrate in 70% and 95% ethyl alcohol.	10 dips in each
6.	Counterstain with eosin-azure 65.	$\frac{1}{2}$ minute
7.	Rinse in 95% ethyl alcohol.	10 dips
8.	Dehydrate in absolute ethyl alcohol.	$\frac{1}{2}$ minute
9.	Clear in xylol.	2 minutes (until clear)
10.	Mount.	

* (From Sachdeva R, Kline TS: Aspiration biopsy cytology and special stains. *Acta Cytol* 25:678–683, 1981.)

After interpretation, most special stains can be decolorized again, and the Papanicolaou stain can be reapplied.

Membrane filter preparations may be made when the clinician is unable to prepare adequate slide films, or when minute tissue fragments, fluid, or blood are drawn into the syringe. The needle with the attached syringe is rinsed with 5.0 cc buffered saline (Hank's solution). This fluid specimen then may be processed immediately or refrigerated for up to 24 hours. After the solution is processed through the membrane filter (we prefer the Millipore filter), the membrane is fixed in a petri dish filled with 95% ethyl alcohol and then stained.

Membrane Filter Stain*

Process specimen; prepare filter:

1.	Fixation 95% ethyl alcohol	2 minutes
2.	Tap water	$\frac{1}{2}$ minute
3.	Hematoxylin (Gill's)	1 minute
4.	Tap water	$\frac{1}{2}$ minute
5.	0.05% of aqueous hydrochloric acid	1 minute
6.	Tap water	$\frac{1}{2}$ minute
7.	95% ethyl alcohol	1 minute
8.	Orange 6	1 minute
9.	95% ethyl alcohol	1 minute
10.	Eosin-azure 65	1 minute
11.	95% ethyl alcohol	1 minute
12.	Isopropyl alcohol	1 minute
13.	Xylol	2 minutes (until clear)
14.	Mount	

* *Note:* Stains change strength, and the timing varies according to usage and storage conditions.

REFERENCES

1. Sachdeva R, Kline TS: Aspiration biopsy cytology and special stains. *Acta Cytol* 25:678–683, 1981.

3

The Prostate and Neighboring Organs

THE PROSTATE

Anatomy and Histology

The prostate is an ovoid organ which resembles a chestnut, and, in men over 50 years old, it measures about $4 \times 3 \times 2$ cm and weighs 20–40 gm. Situated within the pelvic cavity, the gland is surrounded by two capsules, the external or false capsule, composed of extraperitoneal fascia and the posterior fascia of Denonvilliers, and the inner or true capsule; between these two capsules is the venous plexus. The base of the prostate, adjacent to the inferior portion of the bladder, is pierced by the proximal 2–3 cm of the urethra (periurethral prostate). It is bounded anteriorly by the lower portion of the symphysis pubis and laterally by the levator ani muscles. The Denonvilliers' fascia separates the rectum from the gland's posterior surface, 4 cm proximal to the anus. Here the ejaculatory ducts, adjacent to the seminal vesicles, enter the prostate to empty into the urethra.[4] (Fig. 3.1)

The prostate has been divided into areas based on embryologic development, anatomic position, and morphology. A still widely employed classification is the five lobes concept, based on the embryologic development of five distinct solid epithelial buds from the primitive urethra. Since, in the mature prostate, these lobes are anatomically indistinct, and since the periurethral prostatic glands probably originate independently as urethral diverticula, the concept of lobes is being replaced by that of regions.[5,9,14] McNeal[9] identified two zones—the central (inner, periurethral) and the peripheral (outer, subcapsular, cortical)—grossly, with indistinct boundaries but with distinguishing features microscopically. The central zone showed marked arborization of ducts which terminated in elongated sacculations with intraluminal partitions lined by crowded nuclei. The peripheral zone, with less-dense stroma, contained simpler branching ducts and smaller, rounded saccules lined by pale, evenly spaced cells with small, basal nuclei.

17

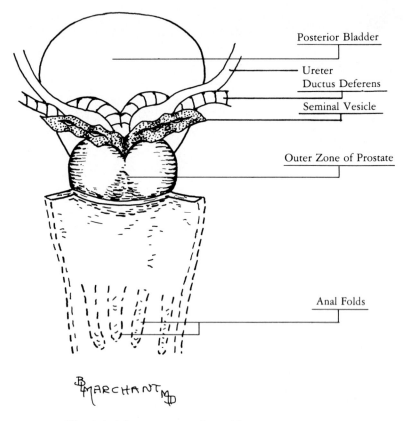

Posterior Bladder

Ureter
Ductus Deferens

Seminal Vesicle

Outer Zone of Prostate

Anal Folds

B MARCHANT MD

Fig. 3.1. The prostate and neighboring organs.

The prostate is composed of 20–30 excretory ducts which extend into the organ from the urethra and open into about 50 sac-like evaginations or alveoli. There also are short glands which drain directly into the urethra.[10] There are two wide, smooth muscle septa, one immediately inferior to the fibrous capsule and the second which surrounds the urethra and separates the central and peripheral zones. Radiating from these septa are smooth muscle and elastic fibers intermingled with collagenous connective tissue which intersperse nerve plexi and capillaries and separate alveoli.

Microscopic sections reveal regularly distributed, elongated or rounded ducts and rounded or oval alveoli, some with papillary evaginations. Most glands are lined by a double row of cells, the basalar, flattened myoepithelial cells and the superficial cells. Moore[12] from study of 678 prostates, described distinct varieties of glandular epithelium. In the active prostate, there are cuboidal, low- or high-columnar, and pseudostratified columnar cells, all coexisting, sometimes within a single acinus. Most numerous are cuboidal and low-columnar cells, with well-defined, homogenous cytoplasm and vesicular or pyknotic nuclei. The pseudostratified cells have granular cytoplasm with indistinct lateral but distinct luminal membranes and oval nuclei; these cells are testosterone-dependent and contain acid phosphatase (see Chapter 7) (Fig. 3.2).

Atrophy of the alveoli and smooth muscle fibers becomes prominent in the pe-

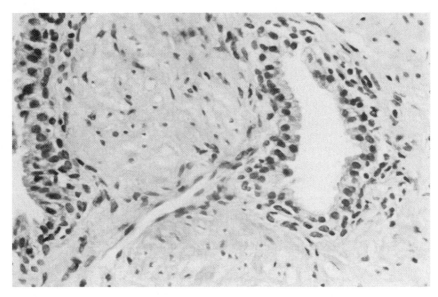

Fig. 3.2. Prostate, histologic section. Note active glands lined by pseudostratified columnar cells. Hematoxylin and eosin preparation. ×300.

ripheral zone.[9] Acini gradually diminish and by age 80, 50% are obliterated. The remainder dilate and are lined by a single layer of cuboidal or flattened, crowded cells (Fig. 3.3). There often is squamous metaplasia of the ducts and increased numbers of corpora amylacea. Smooth muscles are replaced by collagen fibers and connective tissue [see Chapter 4 for aspiration biopsy cytology (ABC)].

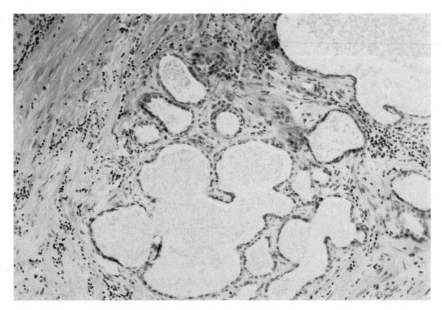

Fig. 3.3. Prostate, histologic section. Note atrophic dilated glands lined by a single layer of flattened cells. Hematoxylin and eosin preparation. ×125.

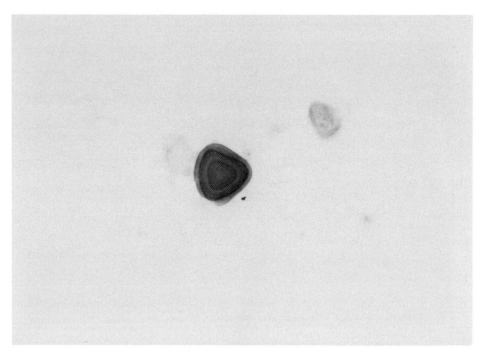

Fig. 3.4. Corpus amylaceum. Note concentric laminations. Papanicolaou preparation. × 300.

Corpora Amylacea

The significance of corpora amylacea (concretions) is unknown. They are unrelated to infection or malignancy, but increase proportionately to age. Originating from prostatic secretions and desquamated cells, they are composed of glycoproteins, and as a nidus may initiate formation of calculi. The concretions, most prominent in the peripheral zone,[11] occupy the lumens of the acini singly or in small groups. In aspirates they are isolated. The spherical or faceted, densely staining, doubly refractile bodies are variable in size, averaging 250 μm in diameter. Their smooth margins and concentric laminations, caused by layering, distinguish the concretions from talc crystals (Fig. 3.4).

SEMINAL VESICLES

The paired seminal vesicles are adjacent to the outer zone of the prostate between bladder and rectum (see Fig. 3.1). Each arises from evagination of the ductus deferens and consists of a convoluted 15-cm tube terminating as a blind sac. On histologic section, branched mucosa rests on a lamina propria of loose connective tissue and elastic fibers surrounded by a thin smooth-muscle layer. The pseudostratified columnar epithelium is composed of a double layer of cells. The superficial, hormone-dependent layer consists of cuboidal or low-columnar cells with vesicular nuclei and well-demarcated cytoplasm containing lipochrome granules. The deep or basal layer has rounded or flattened cells with large nuclei and scant cytoplasm. Sometimes the epithelium contains bizarre cells with poorly defined, scant cytoplasm and hypertrophic, hyperchromatic, irregular nuclei. Arias-Stella,[1] studying seminal vesicle mucosa from 152 patients, noted minor alterations in 35% and marked atypia in 13% of 86 patients over age 45, whereas in the younger men the atypia was nonexistent. These atypical cells, unrelated to benign prostatic enlargement, inflammation, atrophy, or vascular disease, perhaps represent a degenerative or hormone-related phenomenon.[8]

Cells from seminal vesicles are seen in 1–2% of prostatic aspirates, and their occurrence is higher in aspirates from laterally situated nodules. They also appear with increased frequency in aspirates from prostates distorted by previous surgery, radiation, or hormone treatment.[3] These cells are usually few in number and are seen in only one specimen from the two or three passes. They are larger than cells of prostatic origin, measuring 18–25 μm in diameter, and may form mono- or multilayered sheets (see Fig. 9.8), or, most commonly, are isolated. They are triangular or columnar in shape with well-defined cytoplasm containing coarse, yellow-brown lipochrome granules. The single, or occasionally multiple, central, or eccentric oval, bean-shaped, or lobulated nuclei measure 6.2–12.5 μm in greatest diameter and have dense, granular chromatin and occasional macronucleoli. Sometimes there are only bare, irregular nuclei measuring up to 15 μm in diameter. The diathesis is composed of secretions and distorted sperm, either isolated or within histiocytes (see Table 3.1) (Fig. 3.5). In a study of 50 aspirates with seminal vesicle contamination, Koivuniemi and Tyrkkö[7] noted lipochrome granules in 74%, giant

TABLE 3.1. Comparative Cytomorphology—Benign Cells

ABC	Prostate	Seminal Vesicles	Rectum
Pattern	Large monolayered sheets Tissue plugs	Single cells	Small monolayered sheets
Height	7–8 μm	18–25 μm	12–20 μm
Shape	Low columnar	Triangular Columnar	Tall columnar
Cytoplasm	Moderate Secretory granules	Variable Lipochrome granules	Abundant Mucin
Nuclei	Round, oval	Oval, bean-shaped	Elongated, oval
PAP*	Positive	Negative	Negative
Special features	Honeycomb sheets	Bizarre naked nuclei Sperm diathesis	Sheets with peripherally palisading cells

* Prostatic acid phosphatase (see Chapter 7).

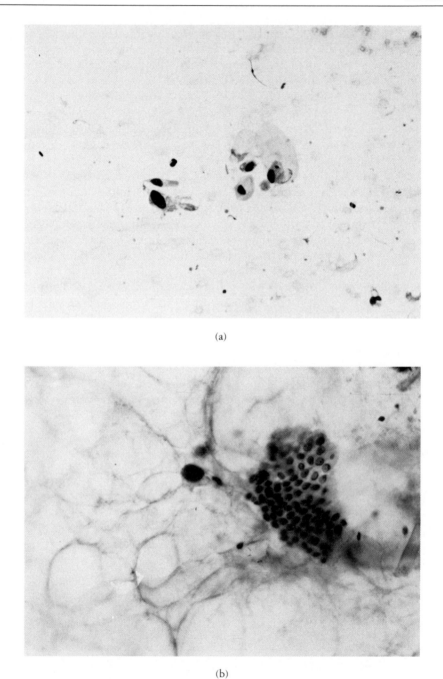

(a)

(b)

Fig. 3.5. Seminal vesicles. **A**. ABC. Note bizarre, isolated columnar and triangular seminal vesicle cells with pleomorphic, hyperchromatic nuclei. Papanicolaou preparation. ×300. **B**. ABC. Note single giant seminal vesicle nucleus adjacent to group of smaller benign prostatic cells. Papanicolaou preparation ×300.

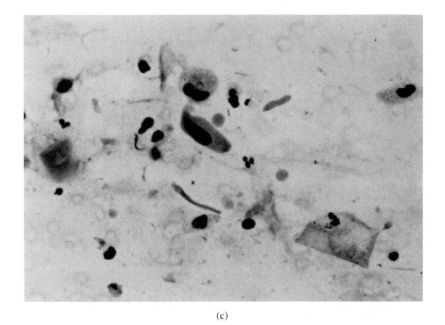

(c)

(d)

Fig. 3.5. C. ABC. Note bizarre cells with cytoplasmic lipochrome and sperm diathesis. Papanicolaou preparation. ×500. **D**. Histologic section. Note epithelium composed of pleomorphic cells. Hematoxylin and eosin preparation. ×300.

nuclei in 66%, prominent nucleoli in 34%, sperm in 44%, and multinucleation in 10% of their cases.

SPECIAL CONDITIONS

Squamous Metaplasia

Squamous metaplasia of the prostatic ducts is found in patients of all ages including the newborn and is associated with a variety of conditions.[15] It may occur spontaneously or with inflammation, infarction, or benign glandular enlargement (see Chapter 4). It is seen 2 or 3 days after infarction[13] and within 3 weeks after the onset of diethylstilbestrol therapy.[2] Microscopically, ducts with metaplastic epithelium, replacing the columnar lining cells, are present in isolated patches or throughout the lobe. The mature, polygonal squamous cells with intercellular bridges partially or completely fill the lumens of the ducts. Cornification of cells has been reported with estrogen therapy.[2]

Cells of squamous origin are frequent in aspirates from the prostate. Intrinsically, they originate from squamous metaplasia of the prostatic ducts, or extraneously from cells of the anal mucosa. Occasionally, foam cells accompany metaplastic cells after infarction or estrogen therapy. Fifty-five men with prostatic carcinoma were examined by NAB after therapy consisting of orchiectomy, hormone therapy, and/or radiation (see Chapter 8). Immature and mature squamous cells were found in the ABC from 52 of 55 patients, unrelated either to therapy or to prognosis.[6]

Squamous cells correspond with those exfoliated from cervical mucosa. They often are isolated but may appear in sheets. Those from the superficial and intermediate layers are large, polygonal, acidophilic, or basophilic cells with pyknotic or small, vesicular nuclei. Solitary, rounded parabasal cells have basophilic cytoplasm and large, vesicular nuclei with dense chromatin. Rarely, there are cells the size of parabasals, adjacent but not in complete juxtaposition with the neighboring cell (pavement formation) with waxy, basophilic cytoplasm and oval nuclei with finely granular chromatin occupying one quarter to one half of the cell volume. There also may be anucleated, hyperkeratotic cells, the size of superficial cells, with hexagonal borders and yellow to orange cytoplasm (Fig. 3.6).

Transitional Cells

Transitional cells appear in less than 5% of the prostatic aspirates. They most often are found in aspirates from small prostates distorted by treatment for carcinoma, and orginate in transitional cell metaplasia of the prostatic ducts (cystitis cystica) (see Chapter 4) or in urethral or bladder mucosa. The cells are larger than those from the prostate, but smaller than cells of squamous origin, measuring about 20 μm in diameter. They may be isolated, in monolayered sheets, or in dense clumps. The cells are oval, faceted, or elongated with central vesicular nuclei

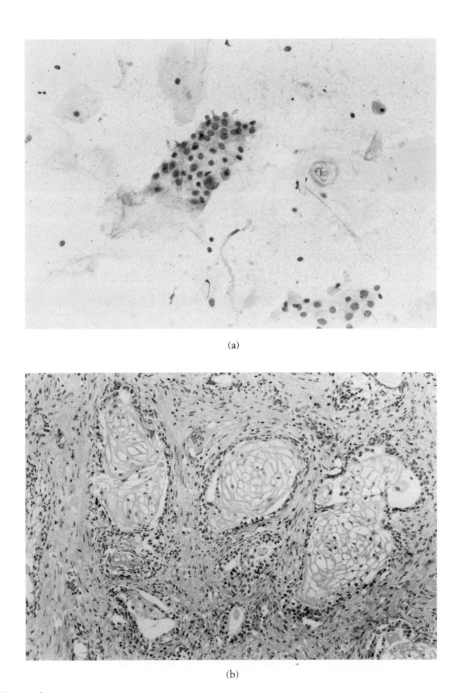

(a)

(b)

Fig. 3.6. Squamous metaplasia. **A**. ABC. Note large, polygonal squamous cells, small oval transitional cell, and central columnar prostatic cells. Papanicolaou preparation. ×300. **B**. Histologic section. Note ductal metaplasia. Hematoxylin and eosin preparation. ×125.

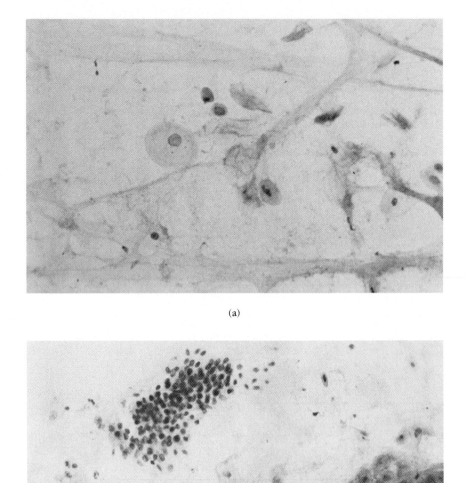

(a)

(b)

Fig. 3.7. Transitional cells. **A**. ABC. Note isolated, small, oval transitional cells adjacent to large squamous cell. Papanicolaou preparation. ×300. **B**. ABC. Note dense groups of transitional cells adjacent to prostatic cells. Papanicolaou preparation. ×300.

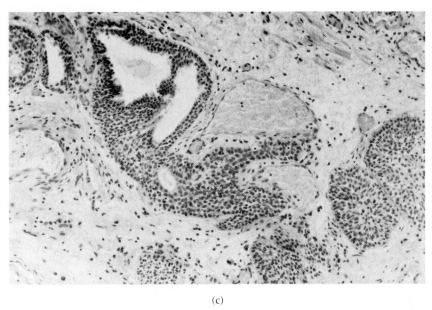

(c)

Fig. 3.7. C. Histologic section. Transitional cell metaplasia (cystitis cystica). Hematoxylin and eosin preparation. × 125.

occupying one quarter to one third of the cell. The dense cytoplasm is amphoteric, with distinctly delineated cell borders (Fig. 3.7).

Rectal Contamination

Rectal contamination is caused by failure to release negative pressure prior to removal of the aspirating needle from the prostate. A few rectal columnar cells are seen in about 25% of the specimens. When rectal cells constitute the bulk of the cell population, the ABC must be interpreted as unsatisfactory. The cells, sometimes accompanied by fecal contamination, are more elongated than most from the prostate. They often are structured in cohesive, well-polarized, monolayered sheets of 30–50 uniform cells with palisading peripheral rows. The cells also may form "picket fence" strips, tightly cohesive cylindrical clusters of 10–15 cells with eccentric nuclei or, occasionally, loose groups of four to ten cells. The tall columnar cells, ranging from 12.5 to 20 μm in height and 2.0–3.75 μm in width, have abundant, granular, well-demarcated cytoplasm. The cytoplasm may be replaced by vacuoles, particularly in cells within large sheets. The eccentric, oval, or elongated nuclei with clumped chromatin, and prominent nucleoli occupy about one third of the cell volume (see Table 3.1). The nucleoli and loose cell groups resembling microacini may suggest well-differentiated prostatic carcinoma. However, a negative immunoperoxidase stain for prostatic acid phosphatase may aid in their true identification (see Chapter 7) (Figs. 3.8–3.11).

Squamous cells from the anus may be present on the ABC. These are indistinguishable from squamous cells of metaplastic origin (see section on Squamous Metaplasia, above).

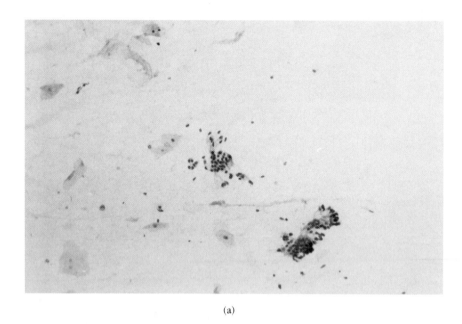

(a)

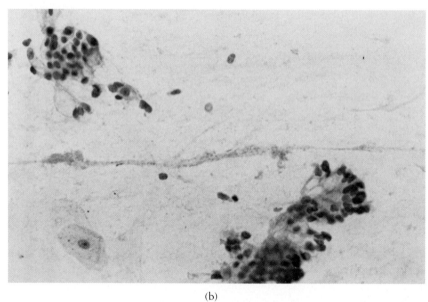

(b)

Fig. 3.8. Rectal cells, ABC. **A.** Note well-polarized sheets with palisading of the peripheral rows. Papanicolaou preparation. × 125. **B.** Higher-magnification view. Note loose cell cohesion. Papanicolaou preparation. × 300.

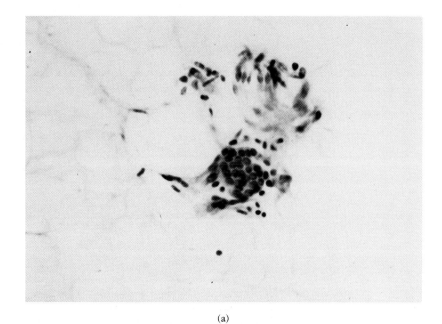

(a)

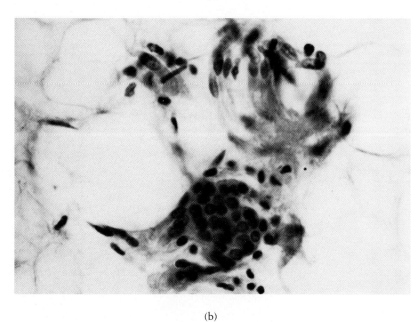

(b)

Fig. 3.9. Rectal cells, ABC. **A.** Note well-polarized cells with peripheral palisading. Papanicolaou preparation. × 300. **B.** Higher-magnification view. Note eccentric small nuclei occupying one third of the cell volume. Papanicolaou preparation. × 500.

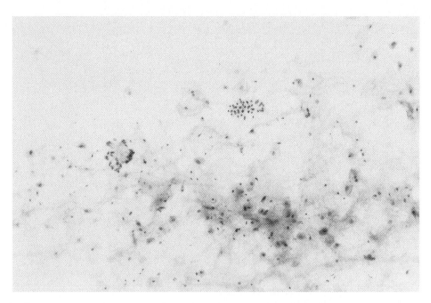

Fig. 3.10. Prostate, ABC. Note pattern of polymorphic benign cells: isolated squamous and transitional cells, loosely clustered rectal cells with peripheral palisading, and cohesive group of small, polarized prostatic cells. Papanicolaou preparation. × 125.

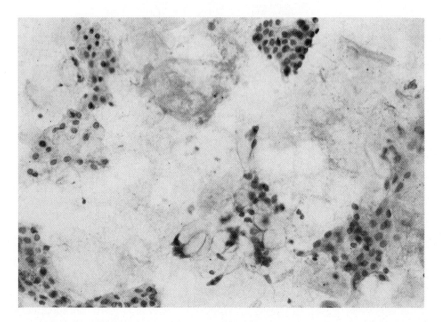

Fig. 3.11. Prostate, ABC. Note structural differences between the central cluster of rectal columnar cells with small nuclei and abundant vacuolated cytoplasm, by contrast to the surrounding clusters of uniform prostatic columnar cells. Papanicolaou preparation. × 300.

REFERENCES

1. Arias-Stella J, Takano-Moron, J: Atypical epithelial changes in the seminal vesicle. *Arch Pathol* 66:761–766, 1958.

2. Bainborough AR: Squamous metaplasia of prostate following estrogen therapy. *J Urol* 68:329–336, 1952.

3. Droese M, Voeth C: Cytologic features of seminal vesicle epithelium in aspiration biopsy smears of the prostate. *Acta Cytol* 20:120–125, 1976.

4. Ellis H: *Clinical Anatomy; a Revision and Applied Anatomy for Clinical Students*, ed 6. Oxford, Blackwell Scientific Publications, 1977, pp. 122–126.

5. Franks LM: Benign nodular hyperplasia of the prostate: a review. *Ann Roy Coll Surg Engl* 14:92–106, 1954.

6. Kline TS, Kohler FP, Kelsey DM: Aspiration biopsy cytology (ABC); its use in diagnosis of lesions of the prostate gland. *Arch Pathol Lab Med* 106:136–139, 1982.

7. Koivuniemi A, Tyrkkö J: Seminal vesicle epithelium in fine-needle aspiration biopsies of the prostate as a pitfall in the cytologic diagnosis of carcinoma. *Acta Cytol* 20:116–119, 1976.

8. Kuo T, Gomez LG: Monstrous epithelial cells in human epididymis and seminal vesicles; a pseudomalignant change, *Am J Surg Pathol* 5:483–490, 1971.

9. McNeal JE: Regional morphology and pathology of the prostate. *Am J Clin Pathol* 49:347–357, 1968.

10. Moore K: *Clinically Oriented Anatomy*. Baltimore, Williams and Wilkins, 1980, pp. 375–381.

11. Moore RA: Morphology of prostatic corpora amylacea and calculi. *Arch Pathol* 22:24–40, 1936.

12. Moore, RA: The evolution and involution of the prostate gland. *Am J Pathol* 12:599–624, 1936.

13. Mostofi FK, Morse WH: Epithelial metaplasia in "prostatic infarction." *Arch Pathol* 51:340–345, 1951.

14. Mostofi FK, Price EB, Jr.: *Tumors of the Male Genital System*. Fascicle 8, Second Series, *Atlas of Tumor Pathology*. Washington, DC, Armed Forces Institute of Pathology, 1973.

15. Saphir O: *A Text on Systemic Pathology*. New York, Grune & Stratton, 1958, pp. 736–753.

4

Benign Prostatic Enlargement

CLINICAL

Benign prostatic enlargement (nodular hyperplasia, glandular hyperplasia, benign hyperplasia, nodular hypertrophy) affects at least 80% of the male population by the age of 80.[4] Both estrogen and androgen have been implicated in its etiology, and it can be reproduced in animals by these hormones. Onset is associated with aging and the presence of testes while regression follows castration. Symptoms, caused by compression on the urethra from encroaching nodules, include faulty micturition, urinary retention, and hematuria. Digital rectal examination reveals smooth, firm, elastic nodules, although differential diagnosis encompasses carcinoma of the prostate or bladder, bladder calculi, chronic prostatitis, or urethral stricture. Surgery is the only effective treatment.

PATHOLOGY

The enlarged prostate averages 100–200 gm[6] but may weigh up to 400 gm with associated infarction.[2] Grossly, the surface is deformed by multiple, well-demarcated nodules bulging into the capsule. These first form in the periurethral area and then progressively enlarge, compressing the urethra and often sparing the outer zone. The nodules vary in size from almost microscopic to more than 2.0 cm. They are gray-white with a firm, whorled surface, yellow-tan and spongy, or partially cystic with milky fluid, Microscopically, there are asymmetrical, nonencapsulated hyperplastic glands, mesenchymal proliferations, or a combination. Dilated or compressed acini are either widely separated by fibromuscular tissue or in close approximation with a few intervening strands of connective tissue.

Glandular (adenomatous) hyperplasia is manifested by an increase in the number of acini and of their lining cells. The glands may show intense secretory activity or signs of atrophy. In the former type, the actively secretory columnar cells evaginate

33

into the lumens to form papillary projections with flattened myoepithelial (basal or reserve) cells along the basement membrane. The columnar cells have eccentric nuclei and homogeneous, clearly demarcated cytoplasm containing secretions. The lumens may be filled with secretions, debris, or corpora amylacea. Inactive (atrophic) compressed or dilated glands are lined by low-columnar or cuboidal cells with scant, ill-defined cytoplasm. Sometimes the glands are lined by a combination of cuboidal and tall columnar cells. Partially obstructed ducts may be dilated and filled with debris and foam cells.

Stromal proliferation (myomatous hyperplasia) is derived from hyperplastic and hypertrophic connective tissue and smooth muscle bundles. The mesenchymal masses resemble uterine leiomyomata but are not encapsulated. In 10% of patients, there may be foci of acute or chronic inflammation or, occasionally, diffuse cellulitis and abscess formation.

Nests of transitional cells (cystitis cystica) may be evident, commonly adjacent to transitional mucosa. These metaplastic foci replace columnar epithelium in the major and minor ducts of the prostate, partially or completely filling the lumens with uniform transitional epithelium (see Chapter 3, section on Transitional Cells).

Infarction is found in about 10% of all prostates and in up to 25% of prostates with benign glandular enlargement.[4] It results from injury to the urethral arteries[5] because of compression from prostatic nodules or from trauma following instrumentation.[2] Microscopically, there are single or multiple areas of hemorrhage, ischemic or coagulation necrosis, or scarring (old infarcts) with peripheral and squamous metaplasia of small ducts and acini (see Chapter 3, section on Squamous Metaplasia).

ASPIRATION BIOPSY CYTOLOGY*

The pattern of benign disease usually is evident by scanning lens. The aspirate is relatively sparse, and there is an orderly arrangement of large, cohesive sheets of uniform cells with intact borders (Table 4.1). There also may be some inflammatory cells, foam cells, histiocytes, squamous cells, and corpora amylacea (see Chapter 3). Epithelial cells from benign prostatic enlargement cannot be distinguished from those of the normal prostate.[1,7]

TABLE 4.1. Criteria of Benignity

Cell paucity
Intercellular cohesion
Sizable, polarized groups
Uniform dimensions of cells and nuclei
Regular nuclear membranes
Distinct cell borders
Cytoplasmic granules

* See Chapter 6, Tables 6.1; 6.2

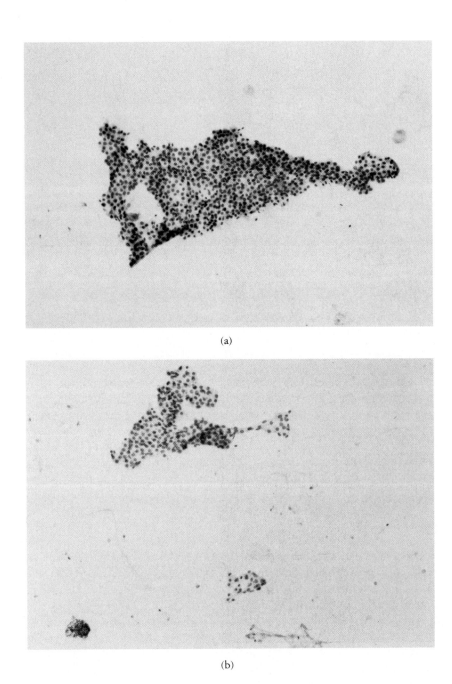

(a)

(b)

Fig. 4.1. Benign prostatic enlargement, ABC. **A**. Note single large cohesive sheet. Papanicolaou preparation. ×125. **B**. Note modest cellularity. Papanicolaou preparation. ×125.

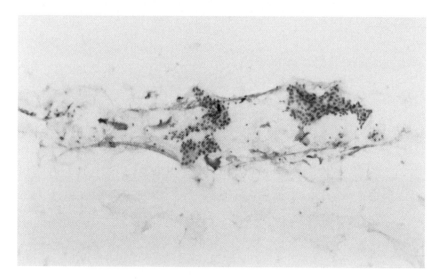

(c)

Fig. 4.1. C. Note relative cellularity; all groups, however, are composed of uniform, cohesive cells. Papanicolaou preparation. × 125.

A cell-poor aspirate is an important criterion of benignity (see Figure 4.1). Cellularity is inversely proportionate to the amount of fibrous connective tissue. In our comparative study,[3] approximately 45% of the benign cases contained one cell group per low-power field, (magnification: 100), and in half these cases there were only two to ten cell sheets on the entire slide. On the other hand, about 10% of the benign cases showed eight to ten groups in a single low-power field. With concomitant infection, cellularity may be intensified (see Chapter 5). What differentiates the scant aspirate procured from fibrotic areas from the technically unsatisfactory aspirate? The interpreter, as part of the team approach to diagnosis of ABC, must know how the NAB was performed; that is, by an experienced operator or a novice.

Benign cells examined under the scanning lens show marked intercellular adherance with regular spatial relationships. Cohesion of cell clusters is judged by compactness, polarity, and peripheral borders which are straight or smoothly rounded. The cytoplasm is clearly delineated, and nuclei are round and relatively equal in size (see Figs. 4.2 and 4.3).

The number of cells comprising each group is meaningful. Groups of 50–200 cells are usually benign (see Fig. 4.4), whereas groups of 3–10 are "suspect". In our comparative study,[3] compact, large, multicellular units constituted the entire specimen in 37% of the aspirates from patients with benign lesions, by contrast to 4% of the aspirates from patients with carcinoma.

The benign cell groups are architecturally variable and gravitate toward three formations: sheets or strips, plugs or fronds, and acini. Most commonly, there are sheets of 50–100 mono- or bilayered, polarized, large cells in honeycomb or mosaic pattern with occasional overlapping of the nuclei. Sometimes, the sheets encircle rounded, secretion-filled lumens, 10–30 μm in diameter (see Figs. 4.5–4.7). Similar cells form well-polarized strips. The individual cells measure 8–11 μm in diameter and have well-defined polygonal or rounded borders. Central, vesicular nuclei with finely granular chromatin and rare chromocenters measure 5.0–5.6 μm and occupy up to half the cell volume. These were the predominant cell type in about half of the cases in our study.[3] Abundant, pale cytoplasm may contain gray-blue, coarse, smudged particles or fine black or yellow perinuclear granules of unknown etiology, not to be confused with the golden lipochrome pigment of cells from the seminal vesicles (see Fig. 4.8). We and others[7] have not observed these granules in malignant cells (see Fig. 9.14).

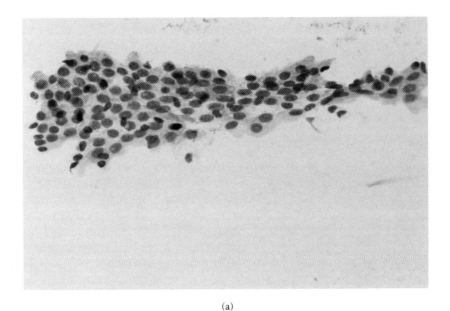

(a)

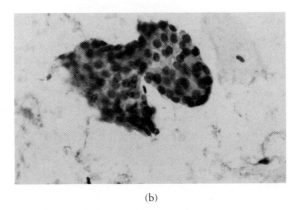

(b)

Fig. 4.2. Benign prostatic enlargement, ABC. **A.** Note large sheet with uniform nuclei and abundant cytoplasm. Papanicolaou preparation. × 300. **B.** Note smaller, polarized cell group with smooth borders. Papanicolaou preparation. × 300.

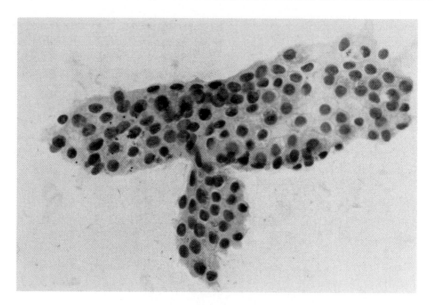

Fig. 4.3. Benign prostatic enlargement, ABC. Note mosaic pattern of polygonal cells with clearly delineated cytoplasm. Papanicolaou preparation. × 500.

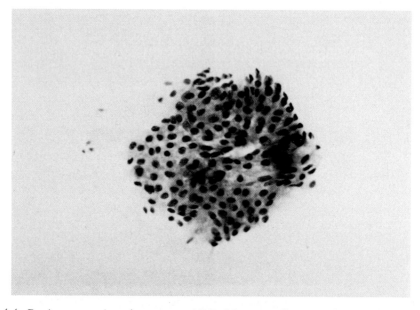

Fig. 4.4. Benign prostatic enlargement, ABC. Note stratification of cohesive, polarized group. Papanicolaou preparation. × 300.

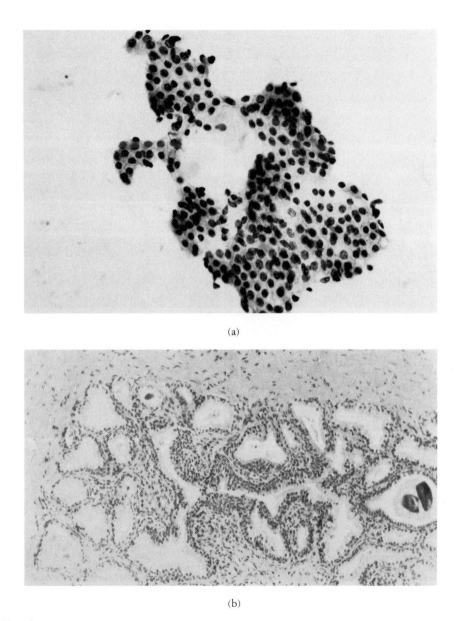

(a)

(b)

Fig. 4.5. Benign prostatic enlargement. **A**. ABC. Note sheet with central lumen. Papanicolaou preparation. × 300. **B**. Histologic section. Hematoxylin and eosin preparation. × 125.

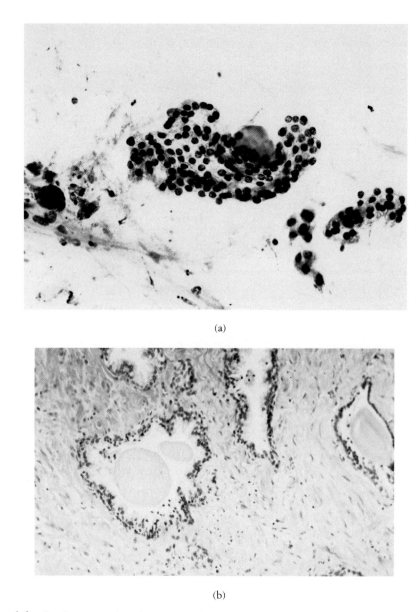

(a)

(b)

Fig. 4.6. Benign prostatic enlargement. **A**. ABC. Note secretion-filled lumen. Papanicolaou preparation. ×300. **B**. Histologic section. Hematoxylin and eosin preparation. ×125.

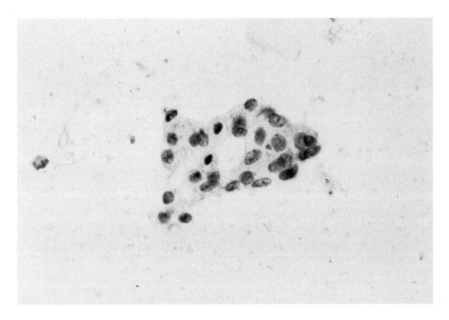

Fig. 4.7. Benign prostatic enlargement, ABC. Note polygonal cells with well-demarcated cytoplasm and central small lumen. Papanicolaou preparation. ×500.

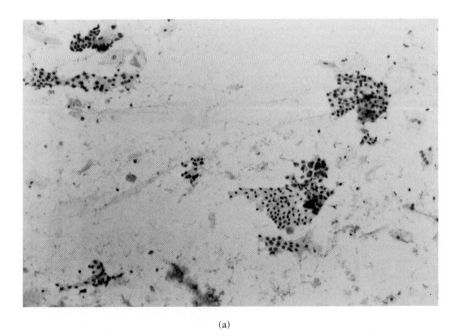

(a)

Fig. 4.8. Benign prostatic enlargement. A. ABC. Note moderate cellularity and cells with cytoplasmic particles. Papanicolaou preparation. ×125.

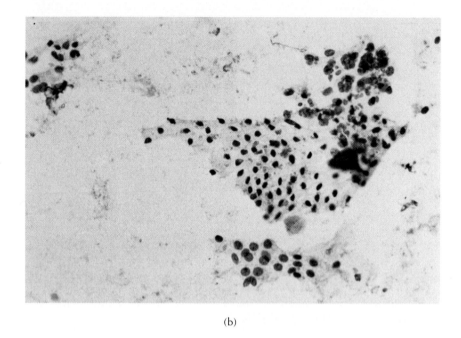

(b)

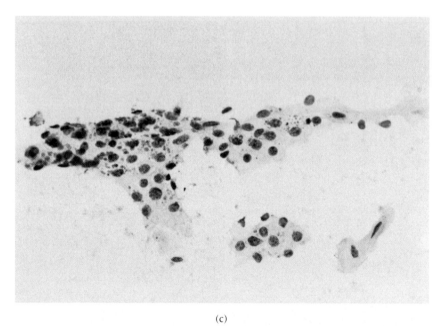

(c)

Fig. 4.8. B. ABC. Higher-magnification view. Note coarse, smudged cytoplasmic particles. Papanicolaou preparation. ×300. **C.** ABC. Note cytoplasmic granules. Papanicolaou preparation. ×500.

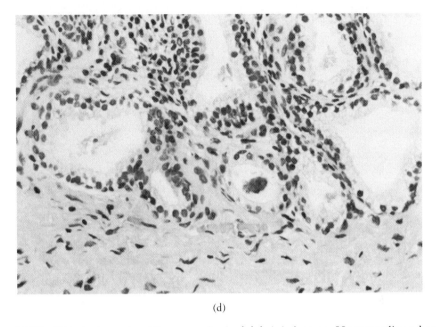

(d)

Fig. 4.8. D. Histologic section. Note secretion and debris in lumens. Hematoxylin and eosin preparation. ×300.

Tissue plugs or fronds, probably originating from atrophic cells, are frequently visible. They are tightly cohesive furls composed of 100–1,000 multilayered small cells. These stratified cells, no greater than 7.5 μm in diameter, have large, hyperchromatic nuclei, occupying about 75% of the cell volume, and scant, ill-defined cytoplasm (see Fig. 4.9).

Aspirates may contain a few acini composed of 5–50 loosely cohesive cell aggregates. These cells, measuring 7–10 μm in diameter, have granular cytoplasm and central or eccentric, large nuclei with dark chromatin and occasional prominent chromocenters. In our study,[3] about 50% of the cases showed a few of these groups. Except for their equal-sized and regular nuclei, they may be mistaken for microacini from well-differentiated carcinoma (see Fig. 4.10) (see Chapter 9, section on Interpretative Traps).

Mesenchymal cells from the stroma are sometimes seen. These well-demarcated strands of cells are composed of interlaced bundles of elongated cells with thin nuclei within a fibrous matrix.

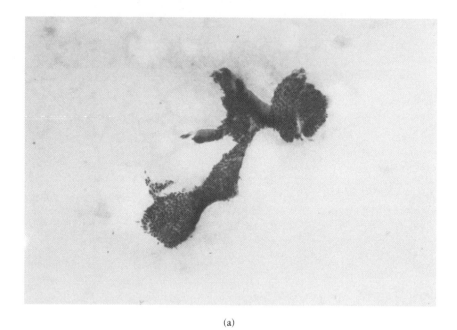

(a)

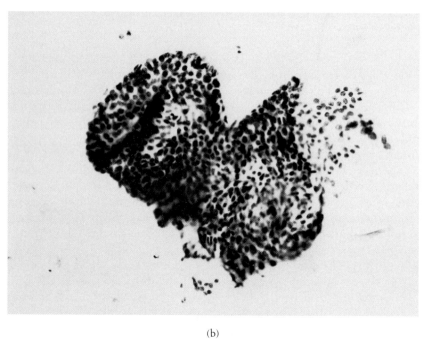

(b)

Fig. 4.9. Benign prostatic enlargement, ABC. **A.** Note frond consisting of about 1,000 multilayered, small cells. Papanicolaou preparation. ×125. **B.** Note cohesive furls. Papanicolaou preparation. ×300.

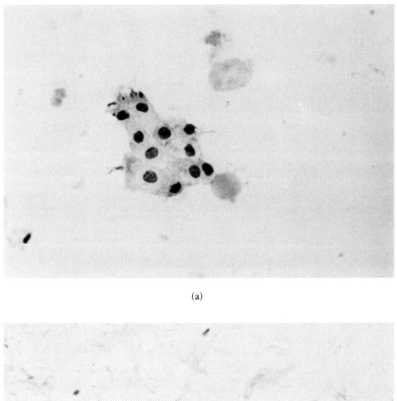

(a)

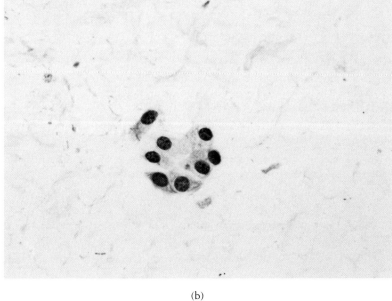

(b)

Fig. 4.10. Benign prostatic enlargement. **A**. ABC. Note cells with small nuclei and abundant, well-demarcated cytoplasm. Papanicolaou preparation. ×500. **B**. ABC. Note formation; these cells may be mistaken for microacini of well-differentiated carcinoma but have well-demarcated cytoplasm and uniform nuclei Papanicolaou preparation. ×500.

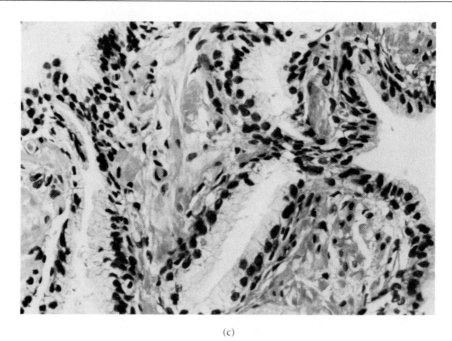

(c)

Fig. 4.10. C. Histologic section. Hematoxylin and eosin preparation. ×300.

REFERENCES

1. Esposti PL: Aspiration biopsy and cytologic evaluation for primary diagnosis and follow-up. In Jacobi GH, Hohenfellner R: *Prostate Cancer. International Perspectives in Urology,* vol 3. Baltimore, Williams and Wilkins, 1982, pp. 71–92.

2. Golden MR, Abeshouse BS: A further clinical and pathological study of prostatic infarction. *J Urol* 70:930–936, 1953.

3. Kline TS, Kannan V: Prostatic aspirates; a cytomorphologic analysis with emphasis on well-differentiated carcinoma. *Diagn Cytopathol* (in press).

4. Moore RA: Benign hypertrophy of the prostate; a morphological study *J Urol* 50:680–710, 1943.

5. Mostofi FK, Morse WH: Epithelial metaplasia in "prostatic infarction." *Arch Pathol* 51:340–345, 1951.

6. Saphir O: *A Text on Systemic Pathology.* New York, Grune & Stratton, 1958 pp. 736–753.

7. Staehler W, Ziegler H, Völter D, Schubert GE: *Color Atlas of Cytodiagnosis of the Prostate.* Stuttgart, FK Schatlauer Verlag, 1975.

5

Prostatitis

PATHOLOGY

Acute prostatitis is caused by a variety of organisms including gonococci, *Escherichia coli*, staphylococci, and streptococci. These bacteria usually spread to the prostate directly from the inflamed urethra but may enter from distant sources through blood vessels or lymphatics. The swollen prostate is often tender, although its firmness may suggest carcinoma. Grossly, yellow streaks may be visible which, microscopically, are abscesses and necrosis. Neutrophils infiltrate acini and edematous stroma. In diffuse prostatitis, the architecture may be replaced completely by the inflammatory exudate.

The prostate affected by chronic prostatitis is enlarged and indurated. The nodules thus formed may be so hard that carcinoma is suspected. In a study of 350 patients with clinically suspicious prostates, 48% had chronic prostatitis.[1] The microscopic image is characterized by infiltration of lymphocytes and plasma cells. There is a proliferation of fibroblasts with formation of connective tissue. Acini, distorted and compressed by scarring, are lined by cells with irregular nuclei and prominent nucleoli. Acute prostatitis may be superimposed on the chronic disease with neutrophil infiltration and abscesses.

Granulomatous prostatitis may be attributable to infectious agents, for example, fungi or acid-fast organisms, but commonly no organism is demonstrable. The etiologic agent may be inspissated secretions or tiny calculi which stimulate formation of granulomas.[5] Palpation of the enlarged, stony nodules gives the configuration of carcinoma. Microscopically, acini are few and are replaced by proliferating fibrous connective tissue and macrophages which may form solid sheets, resembling neoplastic cells.[4] There may be circumscribed, noncaseating granulomas composed of multinucleated Langhans' or foreign body giant cells, epithelioid cells, and inflammatory cells including lymphocytes, a few plasma cells, and eosinophils.

ASPIRATION BIOPSY CYTOLOGY

Aspiration biopsy cytology from prostatitis is cell-dense, sometimes so pro-
nouncedly that the microscopist's initial impression is of carcinoma. The cellularity
is derived not only from inflammatory cells and amorphous secretions but also from
epithelial cells, dislodged from the edematous, inflamed ducts and acini. The atypical
appearance of these cells, partially due to degeneration, disappears following treatment. Specific organisms, including acid-fast bacilli, have been identified on ABC.[6]

Needle aspiration biopsy in patients with acute prostatitis is not usually performed
(see Chapter 1, section on Complications). The cellular aspirate consists of an infiltrate composed principally of neutrophils with a few lymphocytes, histiocytes,
and debris. In addition, there are a few loosely cohesive acini and sheets of columnar
cells with indistinct cell borders. The plump nuclei may have prominent nucleoli
but smooth membranes (Fig. 5.1).

The cell-rich ABC from chronic prostatitis is composed of scattered, atypical
groups of glandular cells, lymphocytes, histiocytes, a few plasma cells, and debris.
The structural arrangement of the epithelium suggests malignancy because of the
disappearance of the honeycomb pattern and dispersal of cells into small clusters
with diminished cohesion. There may be microacini composed of clusters of three
to ten cells shaped into a ring or crescent, with eccentric, variable-size nuclei. In
the medium-sized sheets, there may be some loss of polarity, with nuclear crowding.
The cells have a modest amount of indistinctly-bordered cytoplasm which may contain mucin or secretory granules. The nuclei exhibit anisonucleosis, clumped chromatin, and prominent nucleoli. Eosinophilic nucleoli are rare and nuclear membranes usually are regular (Figs. 5.2–5.5).

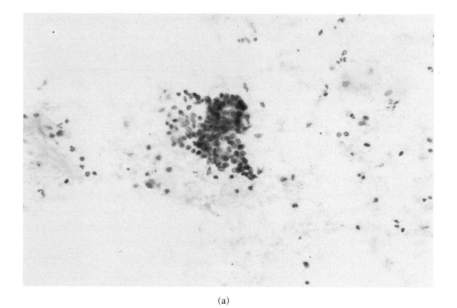

(a)

Fig. 5.1. Acute and chronic prostatitis. **A.** ABC. Note gland with peripheral dyshesion.
Papanicolaou preparation. ×125.

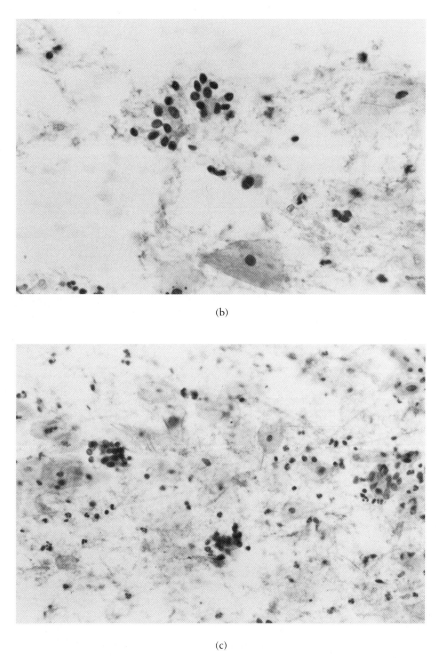

(b)

(c)

Fig. 5.1. B., C. ABC. Note dyshesive small groups resembling microacini with diathesis of neutrophils and lymphocytes. Papanicolaou preparations. ×300.

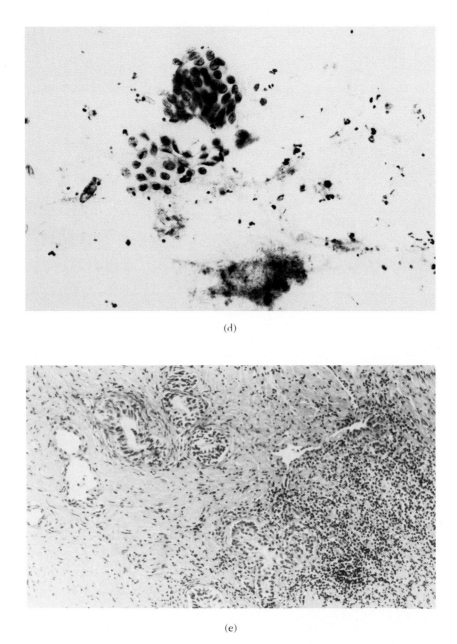

(d)

(e)

Fig. 5.1. D. ABC. Note groups with dyshesion and loss of polarity. Papanicolaou preparation. ×300. **E.** Histologic section. Note acini distorted by inflammation. Hematoxylin and eosin preparation. ×125.

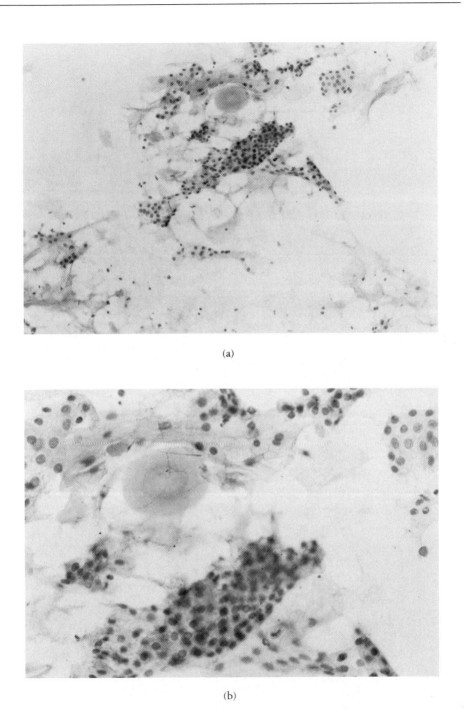

(a)

(b)

Fig. 5.2. Chronic prostatitis. **A**. ABC. Note cell-rich specimen composed of groups with intercellular edema. Papanicolaou preparation. ×125. **B**. ABC. Note partial disappearance of honeycomb pattern. Papanicolaou preparation. ×300.

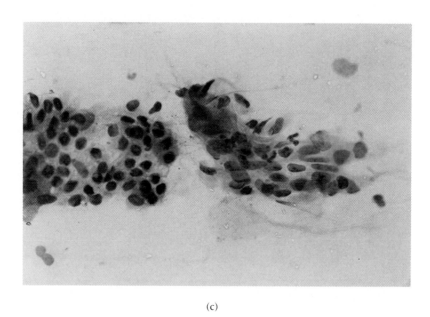

(c)

(d)

Fig. 5.2. C. ABC. Note loss of polarity with nuclear crowding and indistinct cytoplasmic margins. Papanicolaou preparation. ×500. **D.** Histologic section. Note distorted acini lined by cells with loss of polarity. Hematoxylin and eosin preparation. ×125.

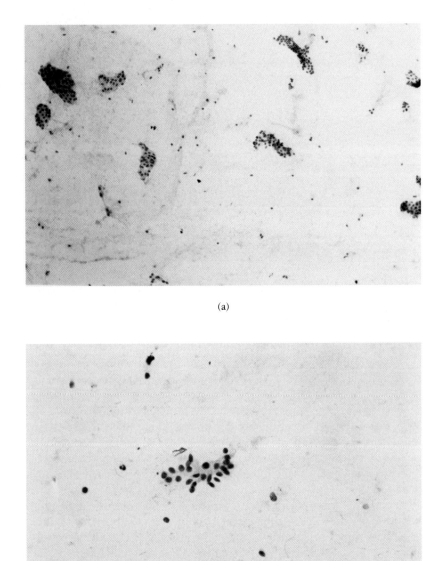

(a)

(b)

Fig. 5.3. Chronic prostatitis. **A.** ABC. Note cellularity with dispersal of some cells into medium and small acini. Papanicolaou preparation. ×125. **B.** ABC. Note small gland with only partial polarity. Papanicolaou preparation. ×300.

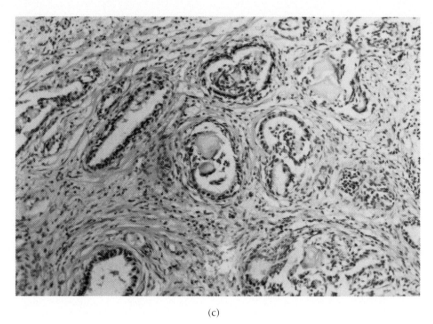

(c)

Fig. 5.3. C. Histologic section. Note dilated acini with intraluminal small cell clusters. Hematoxylin and eosin preparation. ×125.

Aspiration biopsy cytology from granulomatous prostatitis is cell-dense. The epithelial alterations are similar to those of chronic prostatitis but may be more pronounced. Epithelioid cells and histiocytes are present singly or loosely paired with granular, sometimes ill-defined cytoplasm and vesicular nuclei with macronucleoli. The somewhat sparse, multinucleated giant cells measuring up to 75 μm in diameter, have dense granular cytoplasm; the central or peripheral nuclei, often showing anisonucleosis, have clumped chromatin and prominent nucleoli. Kelami and Kirstaeder[2] described the ABC from rock-hard glands of tuberculous prostatitis; groups of cells had abundant but poorly delineated cytoplasm and oval nuclei with chromocenters.

Cell-rich aspirates with degenerated, atypical epithelium and many inflammatory cells must be diagnosed cautiously. Aspiration biopsy cytology from patients with prostatitis often shows some major and minor criteria of malignancy (see Chapter 6) and may be confused with well-differentiated adenocarcinoma. Histiocytes and epithelioid cells may be mistaken for cells from poorly differentiated adenocarcinoma, and multinucleated giant cells with their nuclear variability may be mistaken for malignant acini. Faul and Schmiedt[1] stated that 20% of their first 170 aspirates from patients with chronic prostatitis were erroneously interpreted as suspicious. They recommended that in questionable cases at least eight weeks' treatment with antibiotics should precede a second NAB for definitive diagnosis. Leistenschneider and Nagel,[3] in a study of 129 patients with histologically confirmed chronic and granulomatous prostatitis, differentiated the marked cellular alterations from carcinoma not only by the inflammation but also by the focal nature of the atypia. Definitive diagnosis of malignancy with an inflammatory diathesis must be based only on well-preserved cells with all major criteria of malignancy (Figs. 5.6 and 5.7).

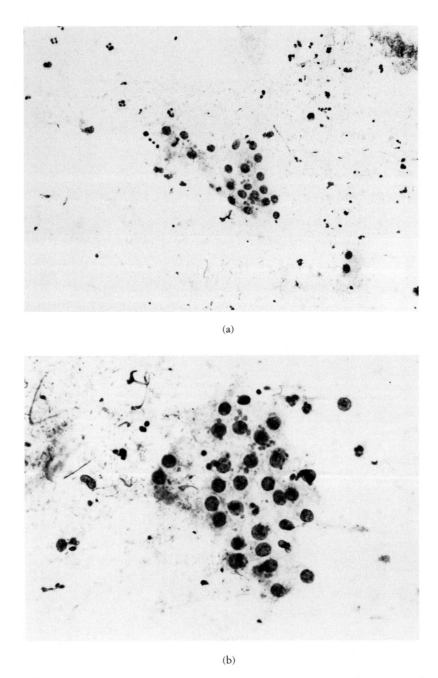

(a)

(b)

Fig. 5.4. Chronic prostatitis, ABC. **A.** Note dyshesive group in inflammatory diathesis. Papanicolaou preparation. ×300. **B.** Note cells with clumped chromatin and cytoplasmic granules. Papanicolaou preparation. ×500.

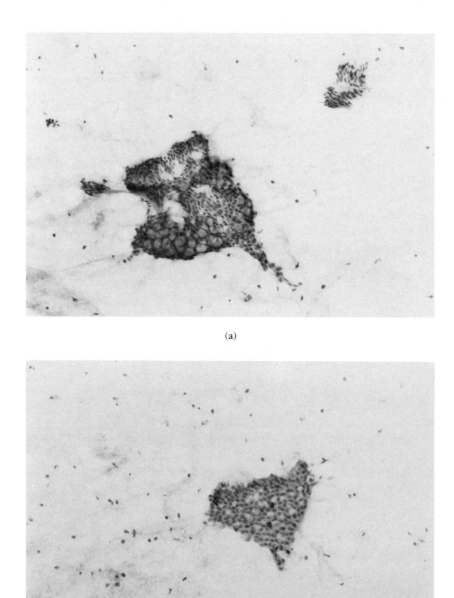

(a)

(b)

Fig. 5.5. Chronic prostatitis, ABC. **A.** Rectal cells. Note cytoplasmic mucin in group with peripheral palisading. Papanicolaou preparation. ×125. **B.** Prostatic cells. Note contrasting pattern between cells with mucin and those of rectal origin in A. Papanicolaou preparation. ×125.

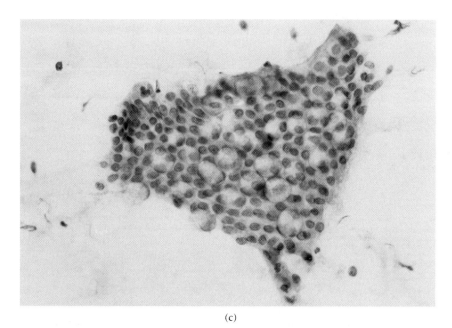

(c)

Fig. 5.5. C. Prostatic cells with mucin, higher-magnification view. Papanicolaou preparation. × 300.

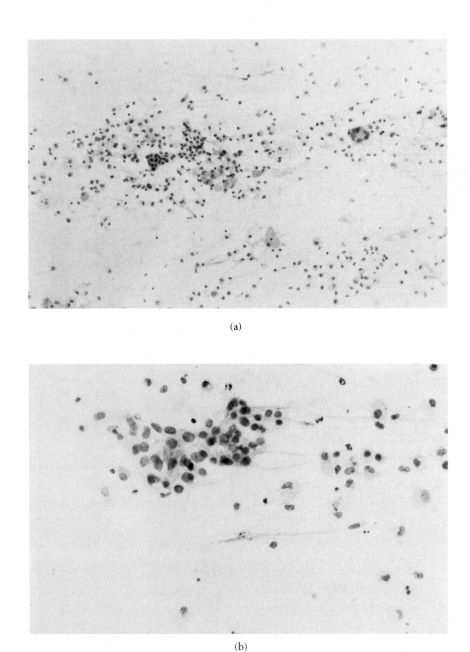

(a)

(b)

Fig. 5.6. Granulomatous prostatitis, ABC. **A.** Note cell-dense ABC with multinucleated giant cell, epithelioid cells, histiocytes, and prostatic cells. Papanicolaou preparation. × 125. **B.** Note dyshesive prostatic cells in inflammatory diathesis. Papanicolaou preparation. × 300.

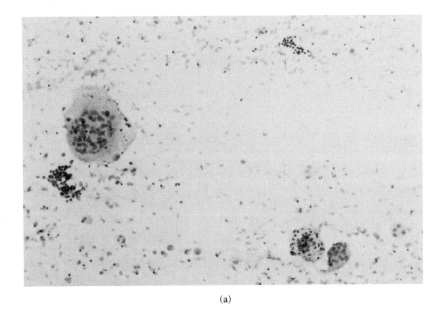

(a)

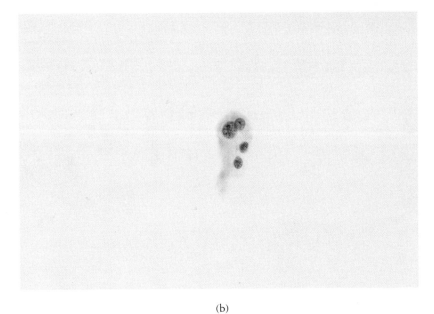

(b)

Fig. 5.7. Granulomatous prostatitis, ABC. **A**. Note huge multinucleated giant cells, by contrast to clusters of small prostatic columnar cells. Papanicolaou preparation. × 125. **B**. Note benign multinucleated giant cell which may be misinterpreted as a malignant acinus because of anisonucleosis. Papanicolaou preparation. × 300.

REFERENCES

1. Faul P, Schmiedt E: Cytologic aspects of diseases of the prostate. *Int Urol Nephrol* 5:297–310, 1973.

2. Kelami A, Kirstaedter HJ: Erste Erfahrungen mit der Franzén-Nadel in der Diagnose des Prostatakarzinoms. *Urol Int* 24:560–568, 1969.

3. Leistenschneider W, Nagel R: Die zytologische Differenzierung der Prostatitis. *Pathol Res Pract* 165:429–444, 1979.

4. Mostofi FK, Price EB, Jr.: *Tumors of the Male Genital System.* Fascicle 8, Second Series, *Atlas of Tumor Pathology.* Washington, DC, Armed Forces Institute of Pathology, 1973.

5. Saphir O: *A Text on Systemic Pathology.* New York, Grune & Stratton, 1958, pp. 736–753.

6. Sparwasser H, Lüchtrath H: Die transrectale Saugbiopsie der Prostate. *Urologe* 9:281–285, 1970.

6

Carcinoma in the Prostate

ADENOCARCINOMA

Pathology

The many classifications of carcinoma of the prostate are beyond the scope of this monograph. Most are based on one of two systems: Mostofi's[23] acinar alterations with cellular anaplasia and Gleason's[14] integration of growth patterns with clinical staging by numerical combinations. It is recognized that about half the carcinomas are composed of areas with at least two patterns of tumor differentiation. Degree of glandular infiltration and invasion of the perineural spaces, lymphatics, or blood vessels are important in some classifications, but the extent of involvement is important in all (see Chapter 8).

Many investigators believe the biological behavior of prostatic carcinoma is related to its histologic appearance. Brawn[4] associated single lumens of variable-sized glands with good prognosis, cribriform or papillary glands with moderate prognosis and sheets, or cords or single malignant cells with poor prognosis. Gleason[13] noted at least partial correlation between grade and stage, and suggested that his system offered "group prediction" and avoided potentially dangerous treatment for neoplasms with low histologic and clinical scores. We diagnose carcinoma according to the glandular and cellular differentiation, stressing the least-differentiated form and indicating its diffuse or focal pattern of growth.

The term "latent" or "incidental" carcinoma is applied to the small, asymptomatic carcinoma found incidentally in a prostate removed surgically or at autopsy. Its incidence ranges from 6.5 to 33% with a marked increase in frequency in men over the age of 80 years.[2,7,15,16,20] Microscopically, the typical pattern is that of a localized neoplasm, present in no more than three microscopic fields, composed of tightly packed, well-differentiated glands without papillations or cribriform formation.[4,24] Disease-free survival is very high, independent of treatment.[2,5,6] Brawn[4] suggested that latent carcinoma carries a low biological potential; he thought this might explain why less than 20,000 individuals die each year of the disease, although 25% of men over age 50 have prostatic carcinoma.

The prostate gland with carcinoma at first is normal in size but later becomes protruberant and nodular, and eventually becomes fixed to its surrounding structures. The firm or stony-hard neoplasm has a stellate shape and greyish-white coloration with yellow streaks.

Diagnosis of well-differentiated adenocarcinoma is based on relatively uniform, mature glandular structures, distinct from adjacent areas of glandular hyperplasia and dilatation. The generally small, rounded, or oval neoplastic glands are clustered back-to-back with little or no intervening stroma or are widely separated and sometimes compressed by dense fibrous connective tissue. The acini are lined by a single layer of low-columnar or cuboidal cells with plump, regular nuclei and prominent nucleoli. There are few or no mitoses.

Moderately differentiated adenocarcinoma consists of an irregular pattern of recognizable glands. The small, medium, or large acini are asymmetrically rounded, slit-like, or have a papillary configuration. The sometimes multilayered cells lining these aberrant glands have less cytoplasm than those from well-differentiated carcinoma and variable-sized nuclei with eosinophilic macronucleoli. There may be intraluminal cribriform or papillary growth.

Poorly differentiated adenocarcinoma exhibits little or no glandular formation. Scattered throughout a fibrous stroma or diffusely infiltrating the normal structures are the pleomorphic glands, irregular cords, or sheets of neoplastic cells. The cells are bizarre, with many mitoses. The cytoplasm may be abundant and vacuolated or barely visible, and the hyperchromatic, irregular nuclei contain eosinophilic macronucleoli.

Aspiration Biopsy Cytology

Diagnosis of adenocarcinoma is based on an altered cellular pattern with the use of ABC criteria of malignancy (see Chapter 1, section on Contrasts and Table 1.1). Dyshesion, an essential criterion, occasions cell density, disarray, and dissolution of large sheets. Nuclear membrane irregularity, anisonucleosis, and macronucleoli are also major criteria of malignancy. Böcking et al,[3] employing semiautomated image analysis and cytophotometry for diagnosis of malignant cells, found significant (in order of importance) the presence and size of nucleoli; nuclear changes—arrangement, anisocytosis, enlargement and polymorphism; and cell dyshesion. Similar to histology, tumor cell differentiation can be ascertained by ABC.[8,11,12] Also, as in tissue sections, well-differentiated malignant cells may be adjacent to moderately or poorly differentiated ones.

The sometimes subtle alterations seen in well-differentiated carcinoma usually can be distinguished from those of benign glandular enlargement by the application of minor criteria of malignancy. These include formation of microacini, enhanced cell size, and nuclear crowding and piling.[19] To ascertain the specificity of these criteria, a retrospective comparative study was made on histologically verified aspirates from 27 patients with benign glandular enlargement, 25 patients with well-differentiated adenocarcinoma, and 20 patients with moderately to poorly differentiated carcinoma.[18] The findings are summarized in Table 6.1, and the conclusions are discussed below.

TABLE 6.1. Cytomorphologic Study—72 Cases

ABC	Benign Enlargement (27 Cases)	Well-Differentiated Carcinoma (25 Cases)	Moderately to Poorly Differentiated Carcinoma (20 Cases)
Groups (×10 magnification)			
2 or more	48%	92%	5%
Rare to 1	52%	8%	95%
Cells per group:			
Small groups (<25 cells)	48%	48%	50%
Large and small	15%	48%	50%
Large groups (>50 cells)	37%	4%	—
Isolated cells	18%	40%	100 %
Anisonucleosis	7%	84%	95%
Macronucleoli	7%	72%	95%
Nuclear membrane irregularity	—	64%	90%
Microacini	—	60%	35%
Nucleus size > 8 μm	—	40%	30%
Cell size:			
<8 μm	48%	16%	15%
8–10 μm	37%	48%	50%
>11 μm	15%	36%	35%
Nuclear/cytoplasmic ratio:			
>80%	15%	36%	45%
66–80%	44%	52%	40%
<66%	41%	12%	15%

Poorly Differentiated Carcinoma

These aspirates display all criteria of malignancy (Table 6.2). The cell-rich specimens consist of small, dyshesive groups with fewer than 25 cells, solitary cells, and naked nuclei. Generally the cells are large in size, at least 11 μm in greatest diameter in a third of the cases in our study.[18] They exhibit poikilocytosis and anisocytosis, and have poorly delineated, moderate in amount or barely discernible cytoplasm. The large nuclei, greater than 7 μm in diameter in half our cases,[18] have irregularly thickened borders and contain eosinophilic macronucleoli. The nuclear/cytoplasmic ratio is also increased; the nucleus occupied most of the cell volume in almost half our cases.[18] In many aspirates bizarre naked nuclei abound. Although these approximate the size of lymphocytes (6–8 μm, in diameter), they are distinguished by irregular membranes, clumped chromatin, and often eosinophilic macronucleoli. For the pathologist or cytologist first examining these aspirates, the diagnosis of poorly differentiated carcinoma is easily made (Figs. 6.1–6.5).

Moderately Differentiated Carcinoma

These aspirates show most characteristics of the poorly differentiated carcinoma (Table 6.2). Indeed, in many cases a number of poorly differentiated tumor cells are intermingled. Malignant cells constitute the majority of the cell-rich population, but there may be a few benign sheets. Tumor cells appear in small, dyshesive fragments, and there are a few isolated neoplastic cells. Naked nuclei are usually absent. Cellular dimensions and nuclear/cytoplasmic ratios are similar to those of poorly differentiated carcinoma. The moderate to scant, ill-defined cytoplasm is granular and without secretions. The central or eccentric nuclei exhibit prominent anisonucleosis, slight irregularity and thickening of nuclear membranes, and macronucleoli which may be eosinophilic (Figs. 6.6–6.8).

Well-Differentiated Carcinoma

The cell pattern of well-differentiated carcinoma may approximate that of benign glandular enlargement (Table 6.2). These cases account for most false-negative and suspicious diagnoses by ABC.[22] The quantity of abnormal cells may be fewer than that from less-differentiated carcinomas, and benign cells predominate. Cell concentration, however, should signal attention to the minor criteria of malignancy.

The microacinus is the most characteristic cellular structure in the aspirate from well-differentiated carcinoma. This is a ring or arc of five to ten loosely adherent neoplastic cells, sometimes exhibiting only slight alterations, including minimal anisonucleosis, nuclear irregularity, and prominent chromocenters. Microacini were found in 60% of our cases.[18] Dyshesion is a significant diagnostic quality that must be analyzed carefully in these aspirates. In our study it was noted in only 48% of our specimens at the initial subjective examination. Yet, when the cells comprising the clusters were tallied, just 4% of these aspirates consisted exclusively of large cell groups in comparison with 37% of those from benign lesions (see Table 6.1). Microacini, too, constitute evidence of dyshesion. In addition, many large sheets show partial loss of the mosaic pattern because of a mild degree of dyshesion. This results in groups with central crowding and overlapping of nuclei and distal scalloping or loosening of cells, by contrast to honeycombed sheets with polarized cells and smooth contours from benign prostatic enlargement. These malignant features must be distinguished from the multilayering of benign cells and are best ascertained by study of peripheral cells for irregular margination and occasional pseudoacinar formation.

The cytoplasm is abundant and secretion-free. Cell borders are indistinct. Anisonucleosis, nuclear membrane irregularity, and/or macronucleoli were observed in most of our cases, but many times they were visible in only a few cells in each specimen.[18]

Enlarged cellular and nuclear size and altered nuclear/cytoplasmic ratio aid in distinguishing the well-differentiated adenocarcinoma from the benign lesion. Often the neoplastic cell is larger than the benign cell; the mean size was 10 μm in diameter in our study. The nucleus also is enlarged and, in almost half our cases, was greater than 7 μm in diameter, by contrast to 5.6 μm in more than 50% of the benign cells. The nucleus occupied more than 75% of the cell volume in 65% of the well-differentiated neoplasms, by contrast to 37% of the benign lesions[18] (Figs. 6.9–6.16).

Infrequently, well-differentiated adenocarcinoma presents a divergent pattern. The aspirate is cell-rich, but the majority of cells are isolated, monomorphic, and larger than other malignant cells, measuring 12.5–18.75 μm in length. The columnar or triangular cells are characterized by eccentric, rather than central nuclei and by abundant but poorly demarcated cytoplasm. The hyperchromatic nuclei, occupying up to half the cell volume, have regular nuclear membranes and occasional nucleoli. They exhibit anisonucleosis, but gravitate toward two distinct sizes, 6.25 μm or 12.5 μm in diameter rather than an intermediate range. Consequently, the nuclear/cytoplasmic ratio averages that of cells from the benign lesion. These neoplastic cells also may be mistaken for benign cells because of their relative uniformity; however, their plentitude should suggest carcinoma. The cells, although resembling those from bladder carcinoma (see section on Secondary Carcinomas, below), are smaller and less pleomorphic than the malignant transitional cells (Figs. 6.17 and 6.18).

In summary, preliminary diagnosis of well-differentiated carcinoma is based on cellularity. With scrutiny, dyshesion is observed with microacini and nuclear crowding and piling. In addition, there often is an increase in cell and nuclear size and alteration in nuclear/cytoplasmic ratio.

TABLE 6.2. Cytomorphologic Features—Summary

ABC	Benign Enlargement	Well-Differentiated Carcinoma	Moderately Differentiated Carcinoma	Poorly Differentiated Carcinoma
Cellularity	++	++++	++++	++++
Number abnormal cells	−	++	+++	++++
Dyshesion	±	++	+++	++++
Anisonucleosis	±	+	++	++++
Nuclear membrane irregularity	−	+	++	+++
Macronucleoli	±	±	±	++++
Microacini	±	++	++	±
Isolated cells	±	*	+	++++
Naked nuclei	−	−		+++
Enhanced cell size	+	+++	+++	+++
Nuclear/cytoplasmic ratio alteration	+	++	++	+++

* Exception—see Figures 6.17 and 6.18.

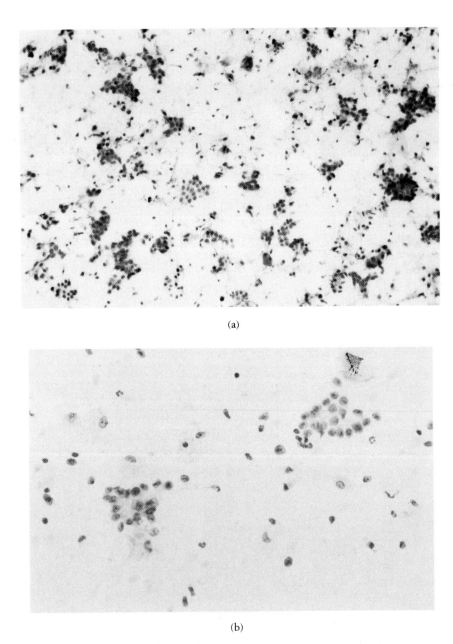

(a)

(b)

Fig. 6.1. Poorly differentiated carcinoma. **A**. ABC. Note cell density. Papanicolaou preparation. ×125. **B**. ABC. Note small dyshesive groups and naked nuclei. Papanicolaou preparation. ×300.

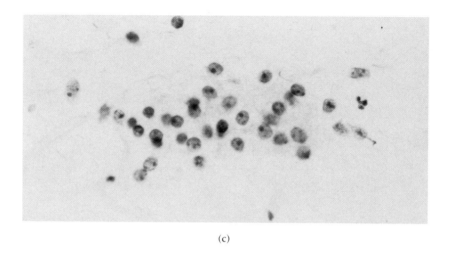

(c)

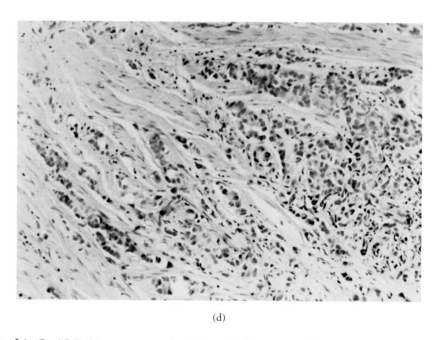

(d)

Fig. 6.1. C. ABC. Note macronucleoli. Papanicolaou preparation. ×500. **D.** Histologic section. Hematoxylin and eosin preparation. ×300.

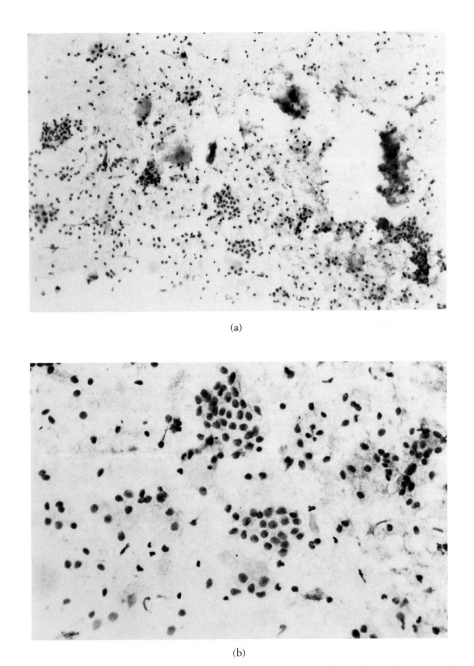

(a)

(b)

Fig. 6.2. Poorly differentiated carcinoma. **A**. ABC. Note cell density with many naked nuclei. Papanicolaou preparation. ×125. **B**. ABC. Note marked dyshesion. Papanicolaou preparation. ×300.

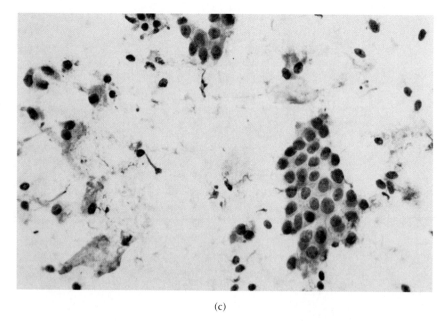

(c)

Fig. 6.2. C. ABC. Note isolated cells. Papanicolaou preparation. ×300.

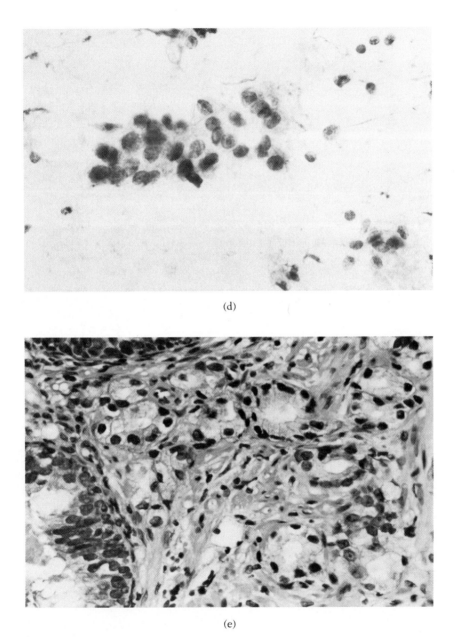

(d)

(e)

Fig. 6.2. D. ABC. Note macronucleoli. Papanicolaou preparation. × 500. **E.** Histologic section. Hematoxylin and eosin preparation. × 300.

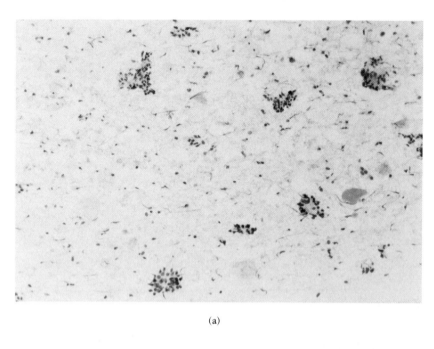

(a)

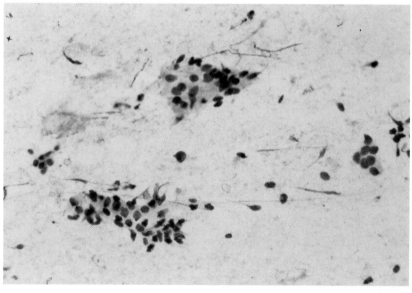

(b)

Fig. 6.3. Poorly differentiated carcinoma. ABC. **A.** Note dyshesive groups and naked nuclei. Papanicolaou preparation. ×125. **B.** Note dyshesive groups. Papanicolaou preparation. ×300.

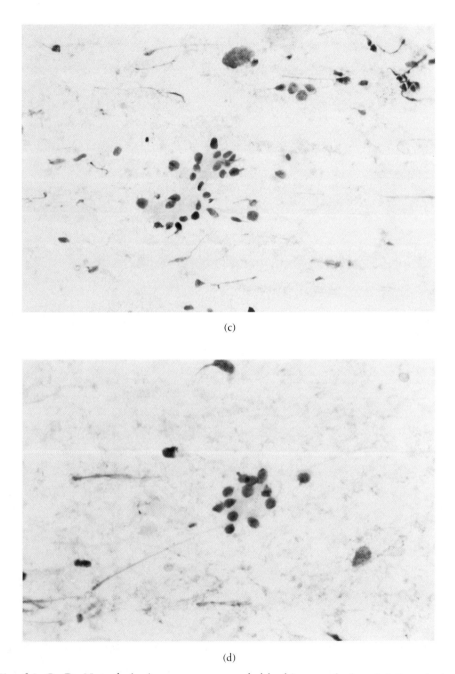

(c)

(d)

Fig. 6.3. C., D. Note dyshesive groups surrounded by bizarre naked nuclei. Papanicolaou preparations. ×500.

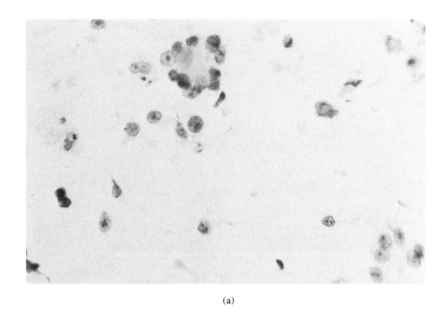

(a)

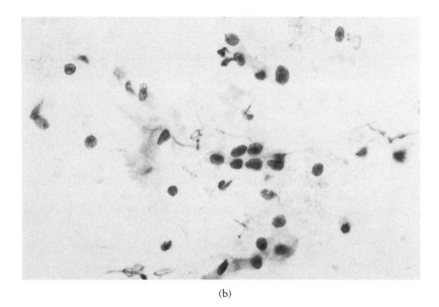

(b)

Fig. 6.4. Poorly differentiated carcinoma. ABC. **A.** Note macronucleoli. Papanicolaou preparation. ×500. **B.** Note large pleomorphic cells. Papanicolaou preparation. ×500.

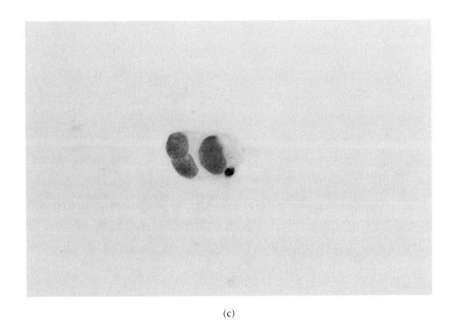

(c)

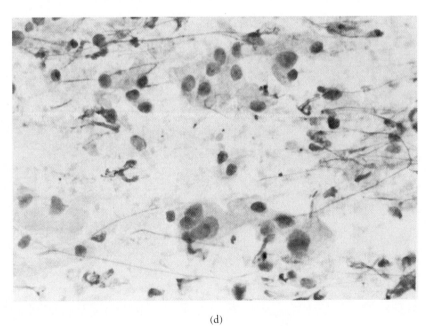

(d)

Fig. 6.4. C., D. Note large pleomorphic cells. Papanicolau preparations. ×500.

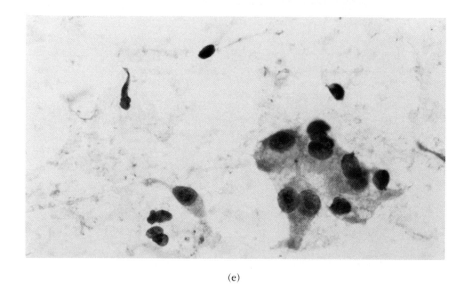

(e)

Fig. 6.4. E. Note large pleomorphic cells. Papanicolau preparation. ×500.

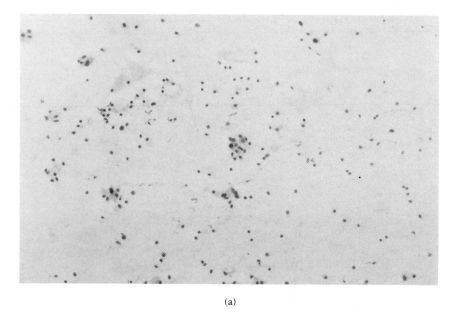

(a)

Fig. 6.5. Poorly differentiated carcinoma. ABC. **A.** Note many isolated cells. Papanicolaou preparation. ×125.

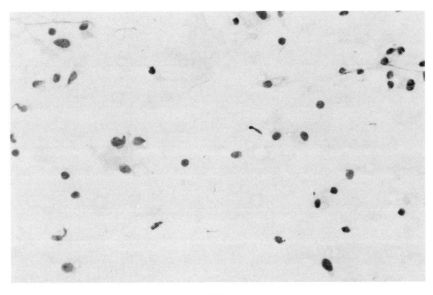

(b)

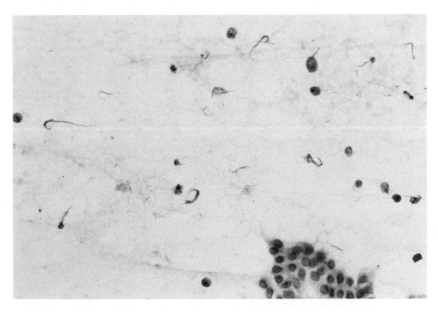

(c)

Fig. 6.5. B. Note isolated cells and naked nuclei. Papanicolaou preparation. ×300. **C.** Note naked nuclei of similar or larger size, in comparison to cells composing the acinus. Papanicolaou preparation. ×300.

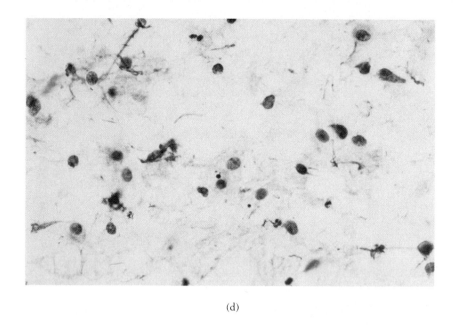

(d)

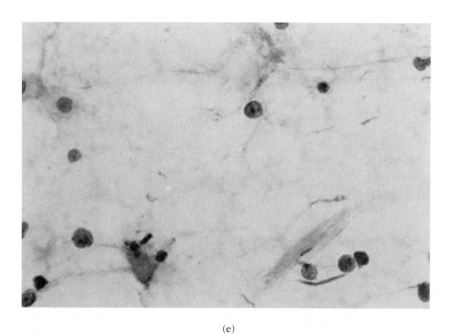

(e)

Fig. 6.5. D., E. Note naked nuclei with some pleomorphism in comparison to the few inflammatory cells. Papanicolaou preparations. ×500.

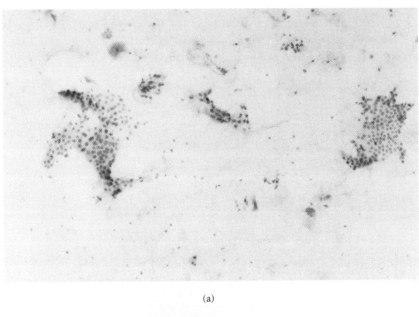

(a)

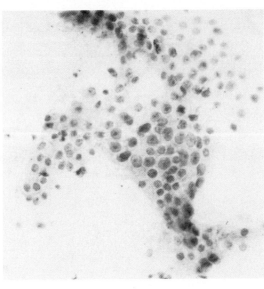

(b)

Fig. 6.6. Moderately differentiated carcinoma. **A.** ABC. Note large- and moderate-sized dyshesive groups. Papanicolaou preparation. ×125. **B.** ABC. Higher-magnification view; note large dyshesive sheet with anisonucleosis and macronucleoli. Papanicolaou preparation. ×300.

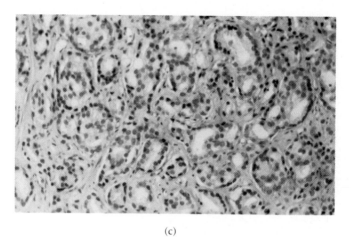

(c)

Fig. 6.6. C. Histologic section. Hematoxylin and eosin preparation. ×125.

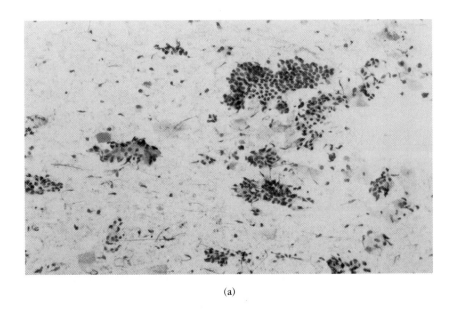

(a)

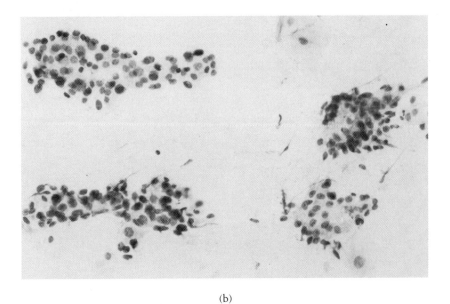

(b)

Fig. 6.7. Moderately differentiated carcinoma. **A.** ABC. Note cellularity and dyshesion. Papanicolaou preparation. ×125. **B.** ABC. Note dyshesive clusters of moderate-sized groups. Papanicolaou preparation. ×300.

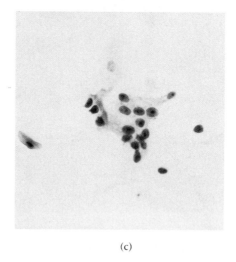

(c)

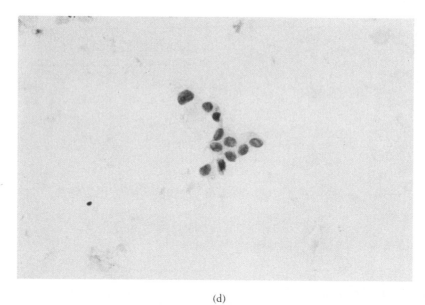

(d)

Fig. 6.7. C., D. ABC. Note dyshesive clusters of small-sized groups. Papanicolaou preparations. ×300.

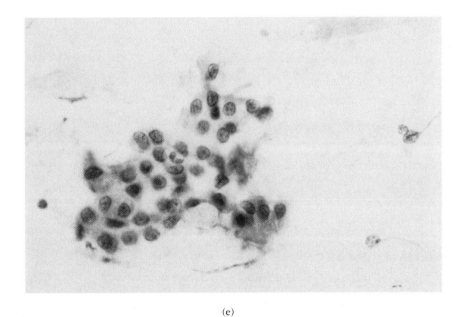

(e)

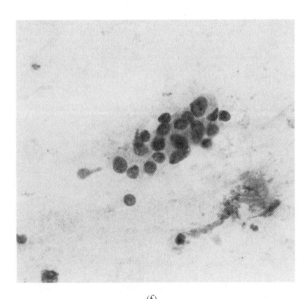

(f)

Fig. 6.7. E. ABC. Note dyshesive cell group with ill-defined cytoplasm. Papanicolaou preparation. ×500. **F.** ABC. Note cells with large nuclear/cytoplasmic ratio and anisonucleosis. Papanicolaou preparation. ×500.

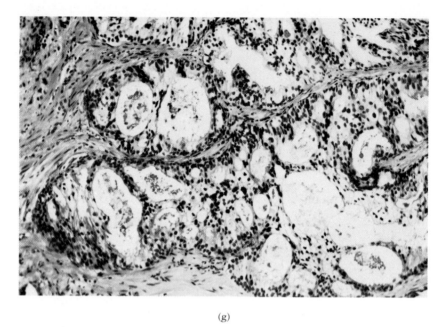

(g)

Fig. 6.7. G. Histologic section. Hematoxylin and eosin preparation. ×125.

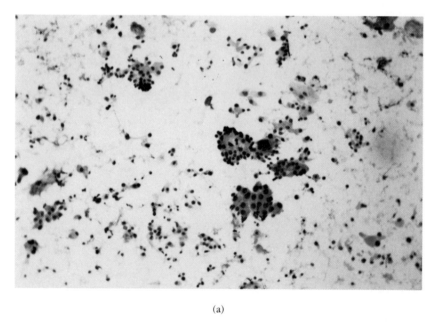

(a)

Fig. 6.8. Moderately differentiated carcinoma. **A.** ABC. Note cell-rich specimen with dyshesive groups and single cells. Papanicolaou preparation. ×125.

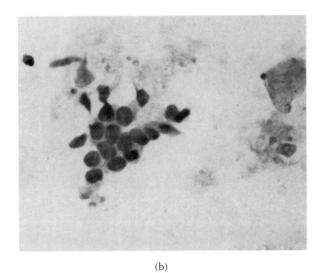

(b)

(c)

Fig. 6.8. B., C. ABC. Note cells with increased nuclear/cytoplasmic ratio. Papanicolaou preparations. ×500.

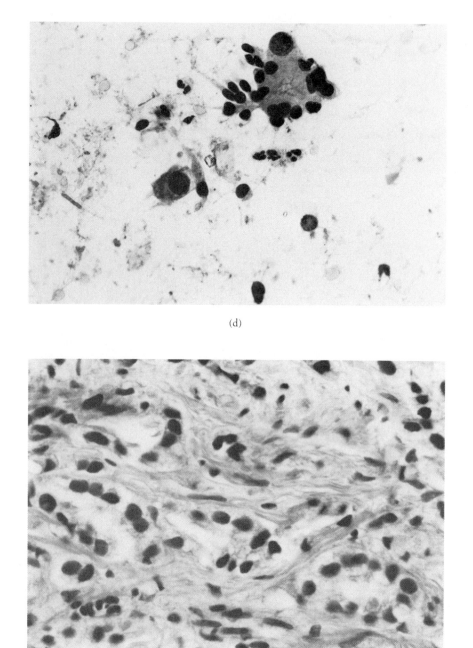

(d)

(e)

Fig. 6.8. D. ABC. Note cells with marked anisonucleosis. Papanicolaou preparation. × 500.
E. Histologic section. Hematoxylin and eosin preparation. × 300.

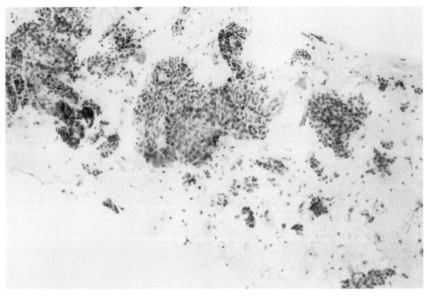

(a)

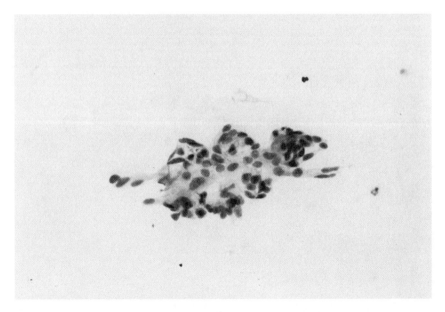

(b)

Fig. 6.9. Well-differentiated carcinoma. **A**. ABC. Note cell density with benign and malignant cell sheets intermingled. Papanicolaou preparation. ×125. **B**. ABC. Note cell group with irregular margination and pseudoacinar formation. Papanicolaou preparation. ×300.

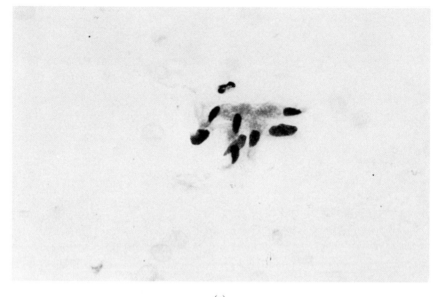

(c)

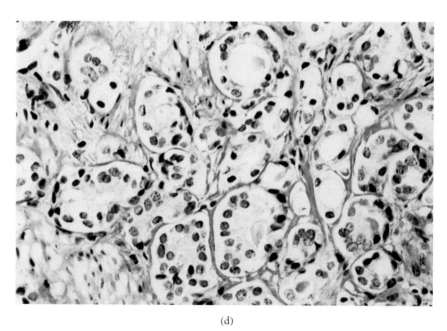

(d)

Fig. 6.9. C. ABC. Note microacinus with slight nuclear irregularity. Papanicolaou preparation. ×500. **D.** Histologic section. Hematoxylin and eosin preparation. ×300.

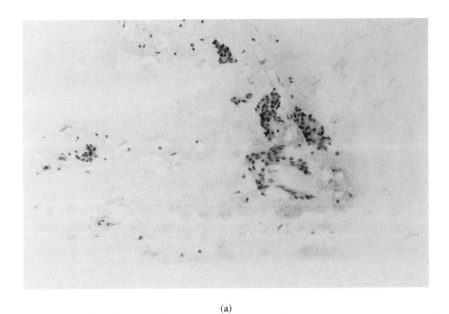

(a)

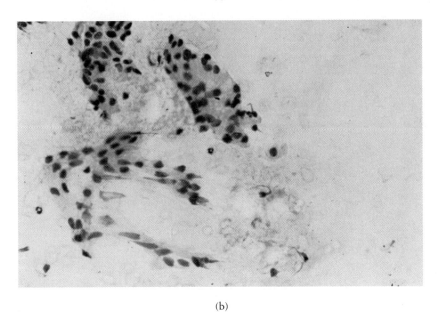

(b)

Fig. 6.10. Well-differentiated carcinoma. **A.** ABC. Note cell concentration and groups with loss of polarity. Papanicolaou preparation. ×125. **B.** ABC, higher-magnification view. Note indistinct cell borders. Papanicolaou preparation. ×300.

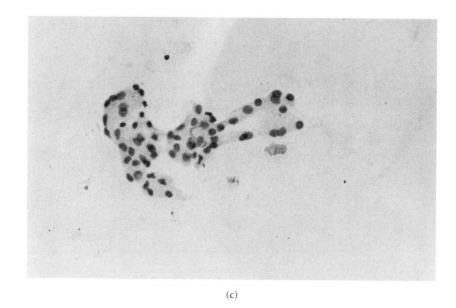

(c)

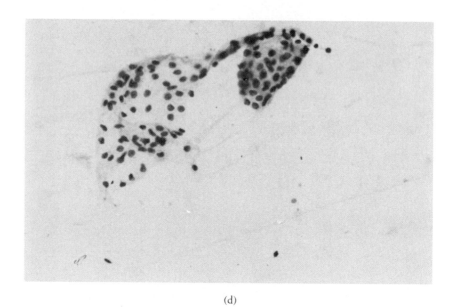

(d)

Fig. 6.10. C., D. ABC. Note loss of polarity. Papanicolaou preparations. × 300.

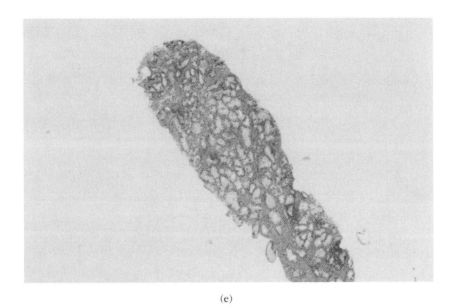

(e)

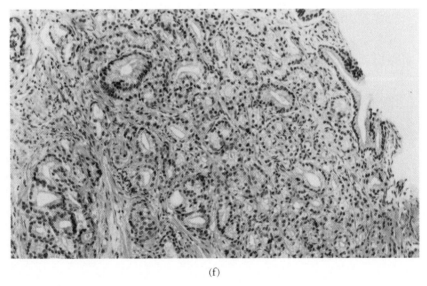

(f)

Fig. 6.10. E., F. Histologic sections. Hematoxylin and eosin preparations. ×30, ×125, respectively.

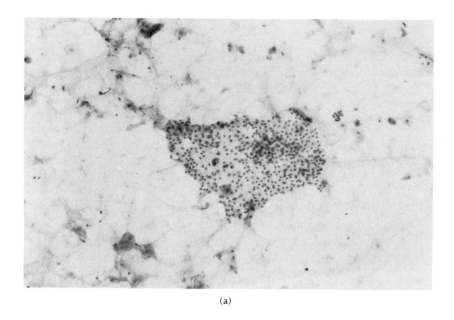

(a)

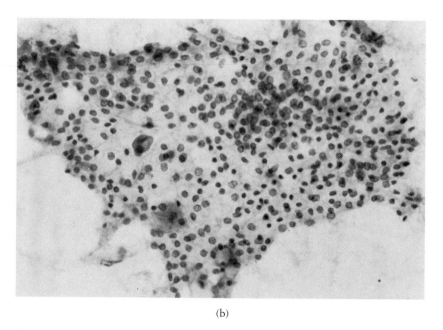

(b)

Fig. 6.11. Benign prostatic enlargement, in contrast. ABC. **A.** Note smooth contours of group of polarized benign cells. Papanicolaou preparation. × 125. **B.** Higher-magnification view. Note multilayering. Papanicolaou preparation. × 300.

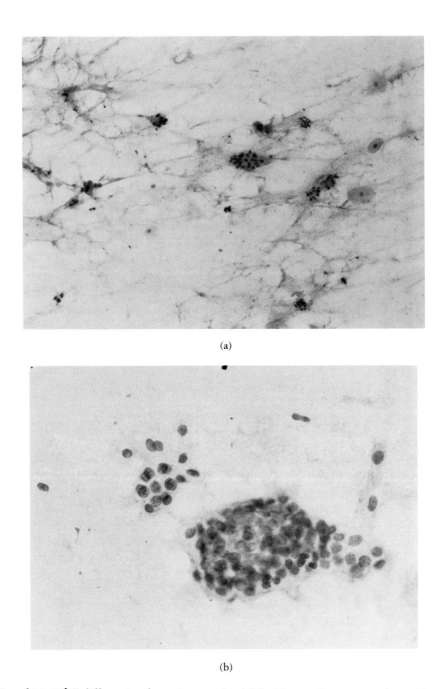

(a)

(b)

Fig. 6.12. Well-differentiated carcinoma. **A**. ABC. Note cell concentration with small groups. Papanicolaou preparation. ×125. **B**. ABC. Note groups with loss of mosaic pattern and polarity. Papanicolaou preparation. ×300.

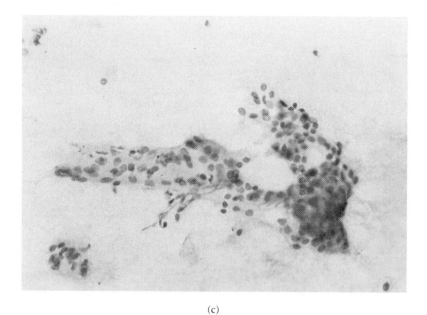

(c)

(d)

Fig. 6.12. C. ABC. Note pseudoacinar formation. Papanicolaou preparation. ×300. D. ABC. Note indistinct cytoplasmic borders and nuclei with prominent chromocenters. Papanicolaou preparation. ×500.

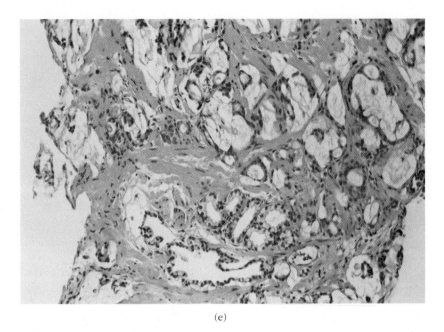

(e)

Fig. 6.12. E. Histologic section. Hematoxylin and eosin preparation. × 125.

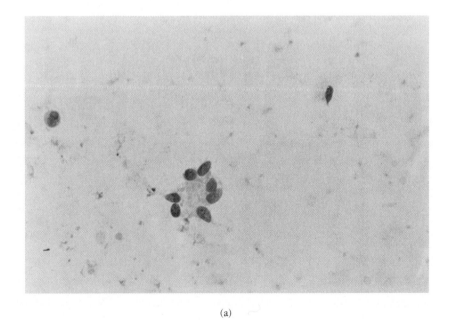

(a)

Fig. 6.13. Well-differentiated carcinoma. **A.** ABC. Note microacinus. Papanicolaou preparation. × 300.

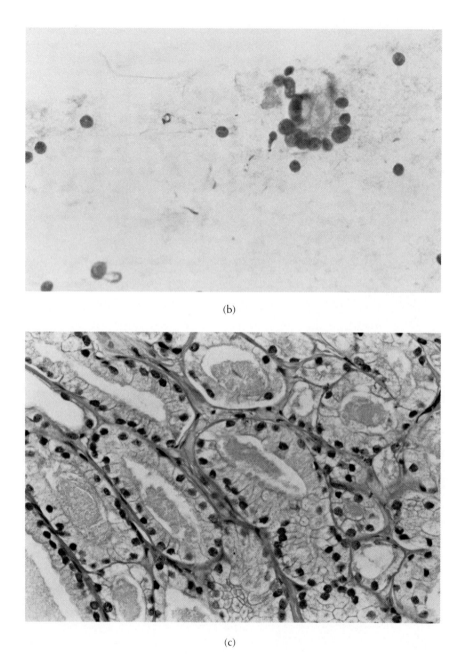

(b)

(c)

Fig. 6.13. B. ABC. Note microacinus. Papanicolaou preparation. × 300. **C.** Histologic section. Hematoxylin and eosin preparation. × 300.

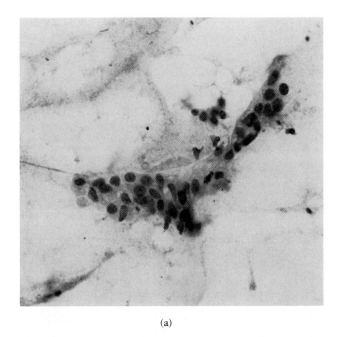

(a)

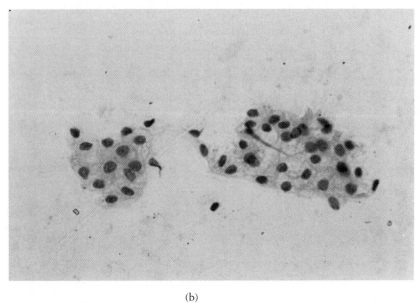

(b)

Fig. 6.14. Contrast ABC. **A**. Well-differentiated carcinoma: Note loss of polarity and indistinct cell membranes. Papanicolaou preparation. × 300. **B**. Benign prostatic enlargement: Note polarity, smaller nuclear/cytoplasmic ratio, and distinct cell borders. Papanicolaou preparation. × 300.

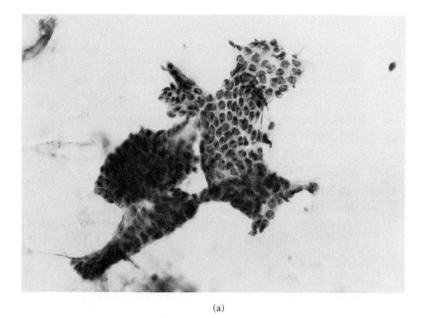

(a)

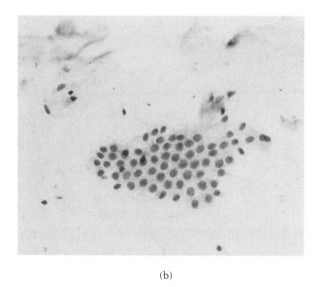

(b)

Fig. 6.15. Contrast ABC. **A.** Well-differentiated carcinoma: Note loss of polarity of peripheral cells with macronucleoli. Papanicolaou preparation. ×300. **B.** Benign prostatic enlargement: Note polarity and smaller nuclear/cytoplasmic ratio. Papanicolaou preparation. ×300.

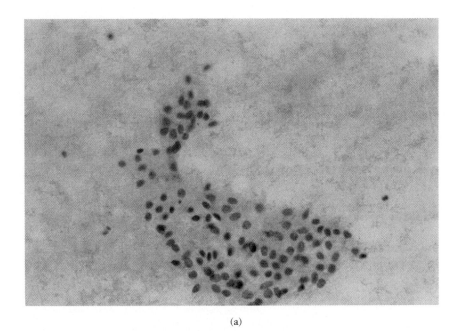

(a)

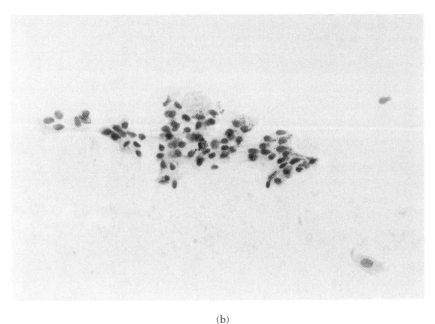

(b)

Fig. 6.16. Contrast ABC. A. Well-differentiated carcinoma: Note loss of polarity and peripheral scalloping. Papanicolaou preparation. ×300. B. Benign prostatic enlargement: Note polarity and relatively smooth peripheral margins. Papanicolaou preparations. ×300.

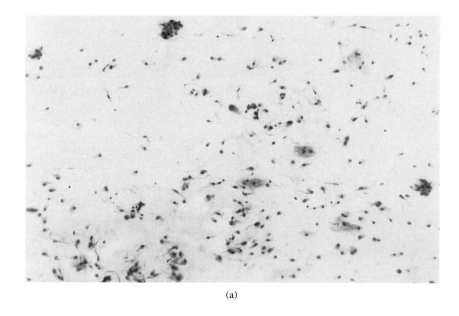

(a)

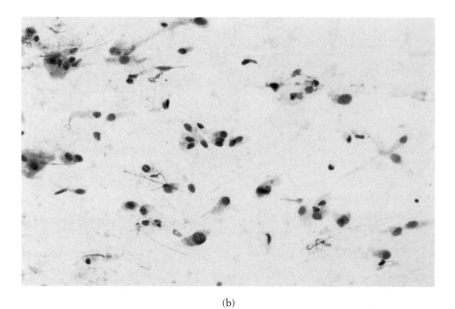

(b)

Fig. 6.17. Well-differentiated carcinoma. **A.** ABC. Note cell density. Papanicolaou preparation. ×125. **B.** ABC. Note columnar cells with eccentric nuclei and abundant cytoplasm. Papanicolaou preparation. ×300.

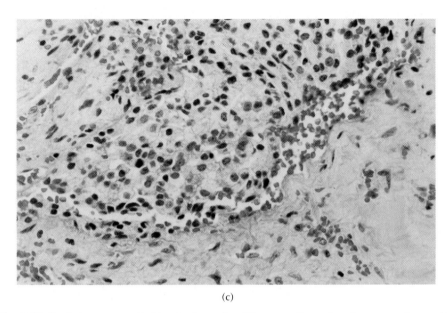

(c)

Fig. 6.17. C. Spine metastasis, histologic section. Hematoxylin and eosin preparation. × 125.

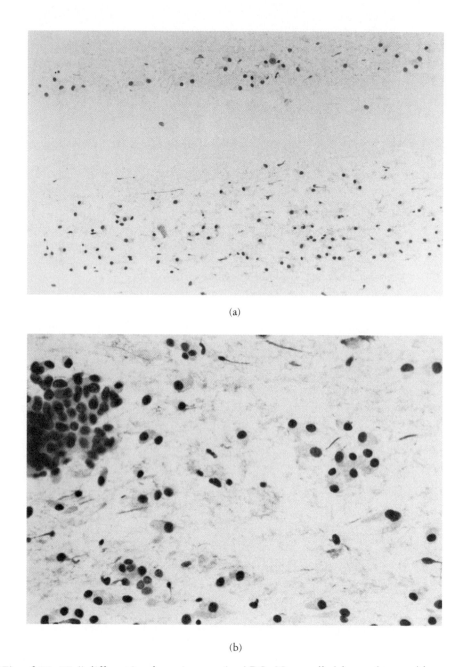

(a)

(b)

Fig. 6.18. Well-differentiated carcinoma. **A.** ABC. Note cell-rich specimen with mono-morphic, isolated cells. Papanicolaou preparation. × 125. **B.** ABC. Note many isolated cells with nuclei occupying half the cell volume and poorly demarcated, abundant cytoplasm. Papanicolaou preparation. × 300.

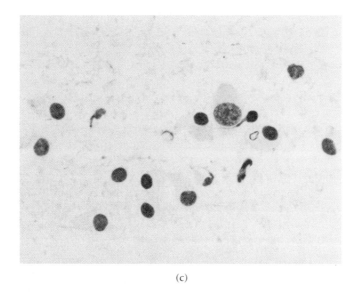

(c)

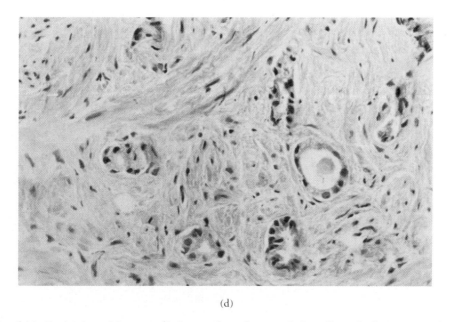

(d)

Fig. 6.18. C. Aspirate. Note two distinct nuclear-size populations. Papanicolaou preparation. ×500. **D.** Histologic section. Hematoxylin and eosin preparation. ×300.

RARE MALIGNANCIES

Mucus-forming carcinoma of the prostate is unusual. The neoplasm is composed of malignant, dilated, mucin-filled acini which blend into non-mucinous areas of prostatic carcinoma.[29] Alfthan and Koivuniemi[1] reported one case with accompanying aspiration biopsy: on initial NAB there were atypical but degenerating cells and much necrotic debris. In a second puncture, malignant columnar cells and signet-ring cells, which gave a positive reaction to periodic acid-Schiff stain, were interpreted as carcinoma of rectal origin. For the correct diagnosis of this rare lesion, immunoperoxidase stain for prostatic acid phosphatase may be useful (see Chapter 7).

Sarcoma of the prostate is very rare, with an incidence of approximately 0.1%. The prevalence is highest in the first decade of life, and 75% are found in patients before the age of 40.[24] Low-grade sarcoma is difficult to differentiate from stromal hyperplasia, and poorly differentiated sarcoma must be distinguished from anaplastic carcinoma. The tumors may grow rapidly, invade the surrounding structures, and produce distant metastases.[27] Müller and Wünsch[25] reported histologic studies with accompanying aspirates from three elderly patients: ABC from one patient, who had a sarcoma with bone formation, revealed a few atypical cells with macronucleoli; ABC from two patients with leiomyosarcomas showed many isolated or loosely grouped, atypical cells with rounded nuclei, rare mitotic figures, and naked nuclei with large nucleoli. The cells from all three cases were easily differentiated from carcinoma by their large size and by the elongation of nuclei with prominent nuceloli; however, these cells resembled the benign pleomorphic cells from seminal vesicles but lacked lipochrome pigment and sperm diathesis (see Chapter 3).

SECONDARY CARCINOMAS

Carcinoma of the bladder frequently invades the prostate. Saphir and Schwartz[28] found prostatic involvement in half the 46 male patients with bladder carcinoma, and noted that the neoplasm metastasized similarly to primary prostatic cancer. Malignant cells from this extracapsular transitional cell carcinoma may be detected by transrectal NAB. These cells customarily are isolated, and are larger and more pleomorphic than the malignant columnar cells from the prostate. The moderate to scant cytoplasm is ill defined, and the central or slightly eccentric, irregular nuceli occasionally contain macronucleoli. Naked nuclei may be present (Fig. 6.19). Malignant transitional cells may be misinterpreted as being from the prostate if there is no history of a bladder neoplasm. Lin et al.[21] recognized the cells from 11 patients as malignant without identifying their source, as well as cells from an additional 3 patients with primary cancer of both bladder and prostate. Esposti[9,10] examined 82 aspirates from patients with extraprostatic carcinoma, chiefly of the bladder, and observed acid phosphatase activity only in the cells from prostatic carcinoma. We studied three cases with transitional cell carcinoma invading the prostate and one with primary carcinoma in both organs, but definitively identified only one which was nonreactive for the antigen by immunoperoxidase technique.[17] Undoubtedly, in future studies, this will be the method for distinguishing the two lesions (see Chapter 7).

Colon carcinoma rarely invades the prostate. Occasionally, however, a carcinoma is pierced by the transrectal needle. We have examined five prostatic aspirates containing malignant cells from the colon; in four, discovery of the primary carcinoma anteceded NAB, but in one it was clinically inapparent (Fig. 6.20):

> A 71 year-old man had a palpable, firm prostatic nodule. Office NAB revealed malignant cells, interpreted as probably arising from the colon. Sigmoidoscopy was performed, and a lesion at 8.0 cm, from the anus, interpreted visually as a papillary adenoma, was biopsied. Histologic section showed an adenomatous polyp, while cells brushed from the region appeared compatible with adenocarcinoma. Core biopsy from the prostate revealed benign prostatic enlargement. A second tissue biopsy from the rectum showed an infiltrating, moderately differentiated adenocarcinoma.

In comparison with cells from prostatic carcinoma, those from colonic carcinoma are generally sparse, although of similar size. They form small, dyshesive, poorly polarized groups or are joined by mucin into relatively cohesive balls of 25–50 cells. These cells have a modest amount of often vacuolated, ill-defined cytoplasm and eccentric, oval, relatively equal-sized nuclei with membrane irregularity and prominent nucleoli. The mucin can be demonstrated by mucicarmine stain[26] (Fig. 6.21).

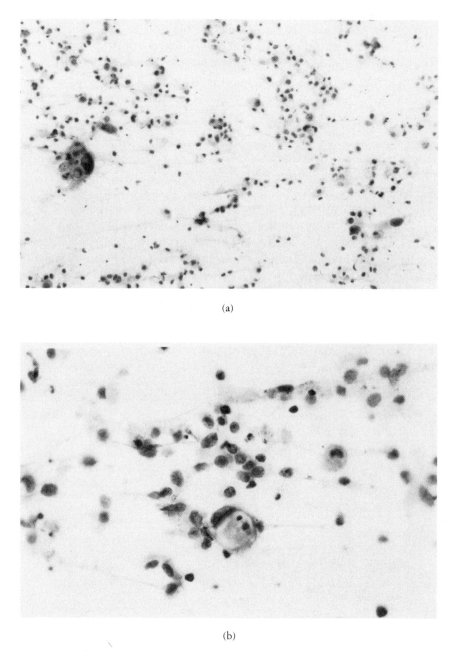

(a)

(b)

Fig. 6.19. Secondary carcinoma from the bladder. **A.** NAB prostate. Note cell-dense specimen with dyshesion. Papanicolaou preparation. × 125. **B.** NAB prostate. Note pleomorphism. Papanicolaou preparation. × 300.

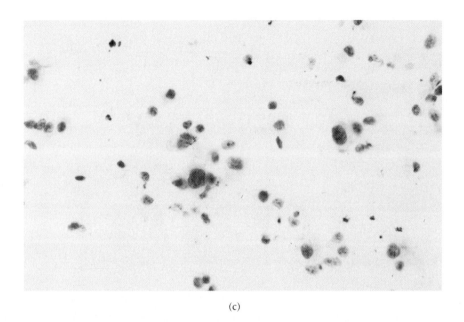

(c)

(d)

Fig. 6.19. C. NAB prostate. Note pleomorphism. Papanicolaou preparation. ×300. D. NAB prostate. Note anisonucleosis and irregular nuclear membranes. Papanicolaou preparation. ×500.

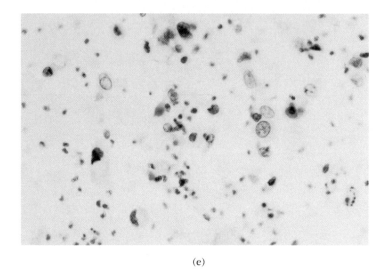

(e)

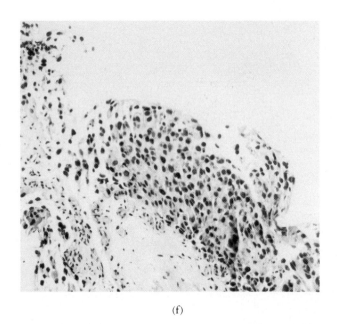

(f)

Fig. 6.19. E. Exfoliated cells, urine. Note similar pleomorphic cells. Papanicolaou preparation. ×300. **F.** Histologic section, bladder. Papillary transitional cell carcinoma. Hematoxylin and eosin preparation. ×125.

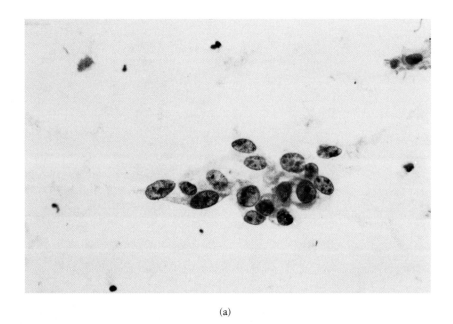

(a)

(b)

Fig. 6.20. Secondary carcinoma from the colon. **A.** NAB prostate. Note dyshesive cell group with anisonucleosis and macronucleoli. Papanicolaou preparation. × 500. **B.** NAB prostate. Note small group with cytoplasmic vacuoles. Papanicolaou preparation. × 500.

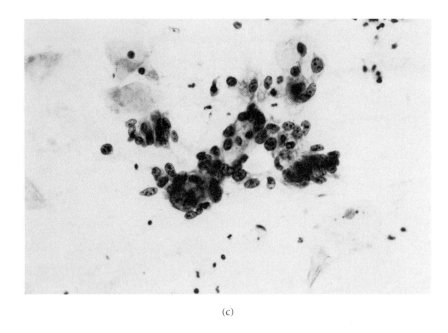

(c)

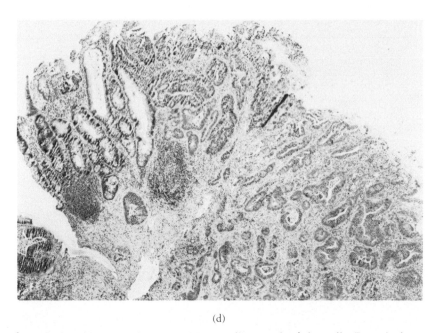

(d)

Fig. 6.20. C. Brushing, rectal mucosa. Note malignant glandular cells. Papanicolaou preparation. ×300. **D.** Histologic section, colon. Note superficial adenomatous polyp with adjacent infiltrating adenocarcinoma. Papanicolaou preparation. ×30.

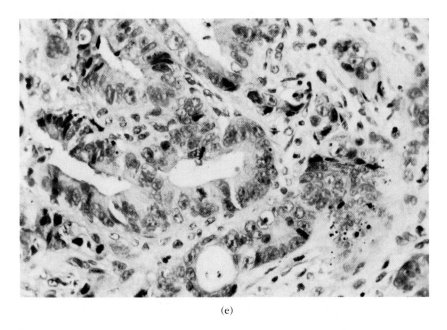

(e)

Fig. 6.20. E. Histologic section, colon. Moderately differentiated adenocarcinoma. Hematoxylin and eosin preparation. × 300.

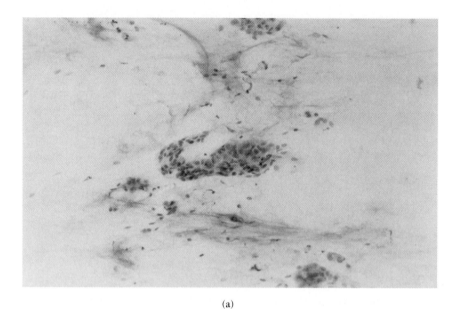

(a)

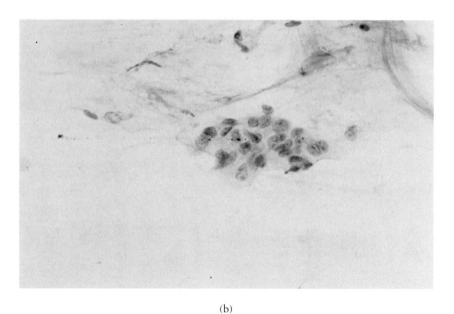

(b)

Fig. 6.21. Secondary carcinoma from the colon; NAB prostate. **A**. Note relatively cohesive cell clusters with mucinous diathesis. Papanicolaou preparation. ×125. **B**. Note cell clusters with loss of polarity and prominent nucleoli. Papanicolaou preparation. ×300.

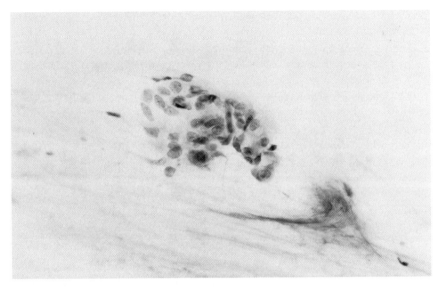

(c)

Fig. 6.21. C. Note cell clusters with loss of polarity and prominent nucleoli. Papanicolaou preparation. ×300.

REFERENCES

1. Alfthan O, Koivuniemi A: Mucinous carcinoma of the prostate; case report. *Scand J Urol* 4:78–80, 1970.

2. Bauer WC, McGavran MH, Carlin MR: Unsuspected carcinoma of the prostate in suprapubic prostatectomy specimens; a clinicopathological study of 55 consecutive cases. *Cancer* 13:370–378, 1960.

3. Böcking A, Auffermann W, Schwarz H, Bammert J, Dörrjer G, Vucicuja S: Cytology of prostatic carcinoma; quantification and validation of diagnostic criteria. *Analyt Quant Cytol* 6:74–88, 1984.

4. Brawn PN: *Interpretation of Prostate Biopsies.* New York, Raven Press, 1983.

5. Byar DP, Veterans Administration Cooperative Urological Research Group: Survival of patients with incidentally found microscopic cancer of the prostate: results of a clinical trial of conservative treatment. *J Urol* 108:908–913, 1972.

6. Correa RJ, Jr, Anderson RG, Gibbons RP, Mason JT: Latent carcinoma of the prostate—why the controversy? *J Urol* 111:644–646, 1974.

7. Edwards CN, Steinthorsson E, Nicholson D: An autopsy study of latent prostatic carcinoma. *Cancer* 6:531–554, 1953.

8. Ekman H, Hedberg K, Persson PS: Cytological versus histological examination of needle biopsy specimens in the diagnosis of prostatic cancer. *Br J Urol* 39:544–548, 1967.

9. Esposti PL: Aspiration biopsy and cytological evaluation for primary diagnosis and follow-up. In Jacob GH, Hohenfellner R: Prostate Cancer. *International Perspectives in Urology*, vol 3. Baltimore, Williams & Wilkins, 1982, pp. 71–92.

10. Esposti PL: Cytologic diagnosis of prostatic tumors with the aid of transrectal aspiration

biopsy; a critical review of 1110 cases and a report of morphologic and cytochemical studies. *Acta Cytol* 10:182–186, 1966.

11. Esposti PL: Cytologic malignancy grading of prostatic carcinoma by transrectal aspiration biopsy; a 5-year follow-up study of 469 hormone-treated patients. *Scand J Urol Nephrol* 5:199–209, 1971.

12. Faul P, Schmiedt E: Cytologic aspects of diseases of the prostate. *Int Urol Nephrol* 5:297–310, 1973.

13. Gleason DF: Histologic grading of adenocarcinoma of the prostate. Short course. International Academy of Pathology 1982.

14. Gleason DF, Mellinger GT, Veterans Administration Cooperative Urological Research Group: Prediction of prognosis for prostatic adenocarcinoma by combined histological grading and clinical staging. *J Urol* 111:58–64, 1974.

15. Harbitz TB, Haugen OA: Histology of the prostate in elderly men; a study in an autopsy series. *Acta Pathol Microbiol Scand* 80:756–768, 1972.

16. Hirst AE, Bergman RT: Carcinoma of the prostate in men 80 or more years old. *Cancer* 7:136–141, 1954.

17. Keshgegian AA, Kline TS: Immunoperoxidase demonstration of prostatic acid phosphatase in aspiration biopsy cytology (ABC). *Am J Clin Pathol* (in press).

18. Kline TS, Kannan V: Prostatic aspirates; a cytomorphologic analysis with emphasis on well-differentiated carcinoma. *Diagn Cytopathol* (in press).

19. Kline TS, Kohler FP, Kelsey DM: Aspiration biopsy cytology (ABC); its use in diagnosis of lesions of the prostate gland. *Arch Pathol Lab Med* 106:136–139, 1982.

20. Liavåg I: Atrophy and regeneration in the pathogenesis of prostatic carcinoma. *Acta Pathol Microbiol Scand* 73:338–350, 1968.

21. Lin BPC, Davies WEL, Harmata PA: Prostatic aspiration cytology. *Pathology* 11:607–614, 1979.

22. Maier U, Czerwenka K, Neuhold N: The accuracy of transrectal aspiration biopsy of the prostate: an analysis of 452 cases. *The Prostate* 5:147–151, 1984.

23. Mostofi FK: Problems of grading carcinoma of the prostate. *Semin Oncol* 3:161–169, 1976.

24. Mostofi FK, Price EB, Jr.: *Tumors of the Male Genital System.* Fascicle 8, Second Series, *Atlas of Tumor Pathology.* Washington, DC, Armed Forces Institute of Pathology, 1973.

25. Müller HA, Wünsch PH: Features of prostatic sarcomas in combined aspiration and punch biopsies. *Acta Cytol* 25:480–484, 1981.

26. Sachdeva R, Kline TS: Aspiration biopsy cytology and special stains. *Acta Cytol* 25:678–683, 1981.

27. Saphir O: *A Text on Systemic Pathology.* New York, Grune & Stratton, 1958, pp. 736–753.

28. Saphir O, Schwarz HJ: Metastases of primary urinary bladder carcinoma invading the prostate. *Arch Pathol* 58:202–206, 1954.

29. Sika JV, Buckley JJ: Mucus-forming adenocarcinoma of prostate. *Cancer* 17:949–952, 1964.

7

Immunocytochemistry

In both ABC and histopathology, specialized approaches may be necessary to determine the tissue of origin of a metastatic neoplasm. In the tissues of a differentiated organism, cells make specialized products which are characteristic of that particular tissue; acinar cells, for example, produce mucin, lymphocytes produce immunoglobulin, and fibroblasts produce collagen. Often cells from a malignant tumor synthesize the specialized product of analogous "normal" cells. The demonstration of these products by their chemical, enzymatic, or antigenic properties can help establish the tissue of origin of the neoplasm.

In the prostate, prostatic acid phosphatase (PAP) is produced by both normal and neoplastic cells. The acid phosphatases [orthophosphoric monoester phosphohydrolase (acid optimum), E.C. 3.1.3.2] are a group of enzymes which catalyze the hydrolysis of esters of orthophosphoric acid and are most efficient in an acidic environment. Acid phosphatases are present in many tissues, including erythrocytes, platelets, bone (osteoclasts), liver, spleen, and the prostate.[16] Multiple enzymes that catalyze the same reaction, yet differ in both chemical and antigenic properties, are termed *isoenzymes*. The biological functions of the acid phosphatase isoenzymes are unclear. In many tissues acid phosphatase is lysosomal and may participate in lysosomal degradation. The prostate-specific isoenzyme, however, is secretory and presumably serves a role in seminal fluid.

Measurement of serum acid phosphatase enzyme activity has been used as a tumor marker since the 1930s, when Gutman and Gutman[12] reported that serum acid phosphatase activity was increased in a high proportion of patients with metastatic prostate carcinoma. To measure serum acid phosphatase activity, an aliquot of serum is incubated with an acid phosphatase substrate in an acidic buffer, and the amount of enzyme activity is measured spectrophotometrically by the rate of appearance of a colored product. The test is limited in usefulness since it measures total serum acid phosphatase activity, rather than the prostatic isoenzyme. Several strategies, utilizing inhibitors and substrates, have been used to measure the prostatic fraction more specifically. L-Tartrate inhibits the prostatic (and other) isoenzymes, but not the erythrocyte isoenzyme.[16] Some substrates are also used more preferentially by the prostatic isoenzyme than other isoenzymes.[1]

Recently, investigators have begun to use a different approach in measuring serum acid phosphatase. The availability of antisera raised against the purified PAP protein molecule allows the use of immunochemical methods[11,27,30] such as radioimmunoassay or counterimmunoelectrophoresis. These techniques measure the presence of PAP antigen without relying on functional enzymatic activity. While the clinical significance of these assays is not yet completely clear,[27,30] the immunologic approach gives greater sensitivity and specificity for the prostatic isoenzyme. However, the specificity of a positive test for the presence of prostatic carcinoma may be lower than that of enzymatic assays, since the more sensitive immunochemical techniques can detect small increases in serum acid phosphatase, perhaps not clinically significant for carcinoma.

The detection of acid phosphatase in histologic and cytologic specimens parallels the efforts in measuring serum levels. Esposti[8] measured acid phosphatase enzyme activity in cells of ABC specimens of prostatic tumors by incubating washed cells in acidic buffer containing substrate and measuring the appearance of product, as one would in a serum specimen. He found that enzyme activity was lower in malignant prostatic cells than in benign cells, but that activity was higher in cells from prostatic tumors than in cells from nonprostatic neoplasms.

Other histochemical approaches have attempted to measure the enzymatic activity of acid phosphatase in cells on glass slides. In this technique, slides holding tissue sections or cytologic smears are overlain with buffer solution containing substrate. Active enzyme in the tissue or cells catalyzes the formation of a colored, insoluble product which precipitates at the site of synthesis and indicates the presence of enzyme activity. Many reaction conditions and substrates have been used for this purpose,[26] and standard techniques exist.[32] Like nonspecific serum measurements, these histochemical techniques measure any acid phosphatase activity, rather than prostatic acid phosphatase alone. Although tartrate inhibition has been used as in serum studies, the results are not totally satisfactory. Phosphorylcholine has recently been advocated as a substrate more specific for PAP[20,31] but needs further study.

With the advent of antisera against purified PAP, the immunochemical measurement of the PAP antigen has become feasible in tissue sections and cytologic smears, as it has in serum. Although a variety of immunohistochemical approaches have been described, they are all conceptually similar. In the first step, high-titered antiserum raised against purified PAP is applied to the slide containing the tissue section or cytologic smear. Antibodies bind at those sites where PAP is present. Antigenic characteristics often survive fixation better than enzymatic activity; thus, the PAP molecule could be enzymatically inactive and yet react with antisera. Since the binding of antibody and acid phosphatase is strong, the specifically bound antibodies remain attached when nonspecific, weakly bound antibodies are washed away. In subsequent steps, antisera raised against immunoglobulin molecules in the first (primary) antiserum are applied. These subsequent antibodies bind specifically only where the primary antiserum has bound and, hence, where there is acid phosphatase antigen. The antibodies in the subsequent antiserum are chemically linked to a marker molecule with either fluorescent or enzymatic properties which make visible the binding of antibody.

Some investigators have reported an immunochemical approach using the fluorescent marker, fluorescein isothiocyanate.[6,13,28] This technique can be performed on either frozen or formalin-fixed tissue and gives high sensitivity and specificity for prostatic carcinoma.[13] However, fluorescent methods require a special microscope, and stained slides cannot be stored due to fading of fluorescence. Immunoperoxidase methods, using the activity of the enzyme horseradish peroxidase as the marker molecule, are more popular because a light microscope can be used, and stained slides can be stored.

The most widely used, highly sensitive immunoperoxidase technique is the three layer peroxidase antiperoxidase technique. The tissue section is first incubated with H_2O_2 to inhibit endogenous peroxidase activity. It then is incubated with normal serum from the same species as the "bridge" antibody (vide infra), which binds nonspecifically to the tissue section, thereby blocking possible nonspecific binding by the subsequently applied antisera. Following pretreatment, the primary antiserum, raised in rabbits against acid phosphatase, is applied and binds to acid phosphatase in tissue sites. After washing, the second or "bridge" antiserum, raised in another animal, such as sheep, against rabbit immunoglobulins, is applied in excess. This binds to the already attached rabbit immunoglobulin molecules. However, since the sheep antiserum is applied in excess, only one of the two antigen-binding sites binds in many antibody molecules; the other remains unbound. After washing, the third layer is applied, a complex of the enzyme peroxidase bound to rabbit antiperoxidase antibodies. The unbound antigen binding sites of the sheep antiserum bind to the newly applied rabbit immunoglobulins, acting as the bridge molecule. Thus, a three layer complex is created: (1) rabbit antiserum binding to acid phosphatase in the tissue, (2) sheep antirabbit serum binding to both layer one and layer three, and (3) rabbit antiperoxidase bound to its antigen. The bound peroxidase retains its enzyme activity. Finally, added substrate (there is a choice of several) is converted to a colored, insoluble product which precipitates at the site of formation, that is, only where acid phosphatase molecules were present in the tissue section.

In every run it is important to include positive and negative controls. A positive control, for example, benign prostatic tissue, demonstrates that the total immunoperoxidase reaction is working. A negative control should consist of the same type of specimen as the experimental sections (e.g., an adjacent section cut from the same paraffin-embedded block or a second smear prepared from the same needle aspiration biopsy). The negative control is incubated in parallel with the experimental specimen, except that nonimmune serum is substituted for the primary antiserum. Since primary antiserum is the only step that is specific for acid phosphatase, the negative control will show only nonspecific binding. If positivity is observed in the experimental section, it is important to verify that the positivity is specific for acid phosphatase by observing a negative reaction in the negative control. If the negative control is also positive, nonspecific binding has occurred, and the positivity in the experimental specimen is not necessarily due to acid phosphatase. We have observed the importance of both positive and negative controls. A commercial kit nearing its expiration date produced weak positive controls and many negative experimental sections. Repeat determination with a fresh kit converted many of the "negative" sections to positive. We also have observed nonspecific binding in histologic sections from papillary thyroid carcinoma and in ABC specimens from breast carcinoma.

The sensitivity and specificity of the peroxidase antiperoxidase technique applied to histologic sections from prostatic carcinoma are high. Nadji et al[23] found that all 37 cases of prostatic carcinoma stained for acid phosphatase, while all 44 cases of nonprostatic carcinoma did not. Although not all studies have reported such perfect results, it is agreed that the sensitivity and specificity of various immuno-peroxidase techniques for primary or metastatic prostatic carcinoma exceed 95%.[10,13,15,17,37,38]

Nonprostatic tumors reported to stain for acid phosphatase have most often been carcinoid or islet cell tumors[10,14] or breast carcinoma.[17,37] The positivity in one islet cell tumor was shown to be due to an enzyme antigenically identical and bio-chemically similar to prostatic acid phosphatase.[5] In breast carcinoma, on the other hand, positivity may reflect cross-reaction with another acid phosphatase isoen-zyme.[9]

The relationship of the degree of positivity in prostatic carcinoma and differ-entiation of the tumor is controversial. While some have found that the proportion of positive prostatic tumors is independent of the degree of differentiation,[4,18,23] others have found that poorly differentiated tumors are more likely to be weakly positive or negative.[3,7,33] It is possible that series finding no correlation between positivity and the degree of differentiation did not include many poorly differen-tiated or anaplastic tumors. Staining is also variable in different areas of the same tumor. Radiotherapy does not appear to lessen production of acid phosphatase within tumor cells,[19] but treatment with diethylstilbestrol (DES) may decrease it.[35]

In comparing various reports on the sensitivity and specificity of immunoperox-idase staining for PAP, it is important to remember that there are many variables. The source and purity of the antigen used to prepare antiserum are crucial. An impure antigen will result in antibody production against the contaminating antigens as well as PAP. The contaminants may be present in nonprostatic tumors and falsely give rise to apparent acid phosphatase positivity. The titer and avidity of the anti-serum and its dilution can affect sensitivity. The type and duration of fixation can affect preservation of the acid phosphatase antigen. These factors may account for many discrepancies in published reports.

While the usefulness of immunoperoxidase staining for acid phosphatase in tissue sections has been extensively explored, little investigation has been made of its potential in ABC specimens. Nadji[21] applied the stain to a few aspirates from pros-tatic carcinoma and concluded that the technique was applicable. We have performed a quantitative study of PAP demonstration by immunoperoxidase technique on ABC specimens.[15]

Aspiration biopsy cytology specimens of primary prostatic carcinoma were cho-sen, retrospectively, from an 8-year period. The slides had been prepared according to the method of Papanicolaou and routinely stored. These cases were compared with ABC specimens of nonprostatic carcinoma and ABC specimens of metastatic prostatic carcinoma.

All slides were stained without decolorization, using the peroxidase antiperoxi-dase technique with commercially available kit reagents (Immulok, now Ortho). The procedure was identical to that outlined in the kit for histologic sections. After examination of the immunoperoxidase reaction, the aspirates could be restained with Papanicolaou stain.

Positive staining consisted of many small, red-colored granules in the cytoplasm. Positivity was unevenly distributed. In large groups of cells, staining often occurred primarily at the periphery; sometimes one end of the slide was strongly positive while the other end was weakly positive or negative. There was usually extracellular background staining, although the acid phosphatase-positive cells were always clearly discernible. Background staining was specific for PAP since it was absent in stained aspirates from tissues not containing the enzyme; the background staining may reflect acid phosphatase antigen released from cells during the trauma of smearing.[21]

To assess sensitivity of the immunoperoxidase demonstration of PAP on aspirated material, we examined a series of aspirates from histologically confirmed prostatic carcinoma (Table 7.1). Of 28 cases of moderately or poorly differentiated prostatic carcinoma, 27 were positive for PAP. Although not each malignant cell stained, many positive cells were distributed over the slide. In 18 of these cases with an additional available slide, a parallel incubation with nonimmune primary antiserum was negative, confirming the reaction specificity for PAP. Histologic specimens (chiefly core-needle biopsies) from 16 of 17 cases were positive for PAP, all confirmed by substitution of primary antiserum; the single negative specimen was the same case which was negative for PAP in the aspirate. Seventeen of 18 ABC specimens and 18 accompanying histologic specimens from well-differentiated prostatic carcinoma were positive. The single nonreacting aspirate contained positively stained benign cells, serving as an internal control.

Thus, we observed sensitivity for PAP in tissue sections of prostatic carcinoma in the same range as that reported by others. Furthermore, the sensitivity of the reaction in aspirates is virtually identical to the high sensitivity seen in tissue sections. In our series, the degree of differentiation of the tumor did not affect the proportion of positive cases, although staining did appear lighter or more focal in some of the moderately and/or poorly differentiated carcinomas. Similarly, there was no consistent difference in staining pattern between benign and malignant prostatic cells. Thus, the reaction cannot be used to establish the presence of a malignant tumor, but only to indicate the prostatic origin of the cells.

The immunoperoxidase reaction could be performed on both recent and older aspirates. Fourteen ABC specimens of prostatic carcinoma were taken at least 4 years earlier, and one was 8 years old, with no difference in reactivity. Thus, the immunoperoxidase technique shows good sensitivity on ABC specimens from primary prostatic carcinoma, with antigenic reactivity maintained for at least 8 years of storage.

There were four ABC specimens from patients with proven metastatic prostatic carcinoma. Two were from lymph nodes (cervical and supraclavicular), one was from a peripancreatic mass, and one was prepared at autopsy from a dural metastasis. All

TABLE 7.1. Prostatic Acid Phosphatase Positivity in Prostatic Carcinoma

Carcinoma	ABC		Histology	
Primary, moderately to poorly differentiated	27/28	(96%)*	16/17	(94%)
Primary, well differentiated	17/18	(94%)	18/18	(100%)
Metastases	4/4	(100%)	1/1	

* Ratio of positive to total cases.

four were diffusely positive for PAP by immunoperoxidase technique (see Table 7.1), showing that the antigen can be demonstrated in ABC specimens of metastatic, as well as primary, prostatic carcinoma (Plates 1–6) (see also Figs. 9.8–9.10).

To evaluate the specificity for prostatic carcinoma of PAP stained by immuno-peroxidase, we investigated ABC specimens from 21 primary or metastatic tumors of nonprostatic origin, including lung, breast, colon, and pancreas. Only two spec-imens, both from patients with infiltrating ductal carcinoma of the breast, were positive, showing reactivity in only two or three cells per slide (Table 7.2); the corresponding histologic sections of the breast tumors stained negatively for PAP. The specificity of the technique also was demonstrated by a negative reaction on a prostatic ABC specimen with malignant cells which could have originated from either a primary prostatic carcinoma or bladder carcinoma invading the prostate (see Chapter 6, section on Secondary Carcinomas). The PAP negativity suggested a primary bladder carcinoma, which was subsequently confirmed by bladder biopsy.

Validation of high sensitivity and specificity for the immunochemical demon-stration of PAP in ABC specimens means that the assay can be used on aspirates as it is in histologic specimens, to elucidate the tissue of origin of a neoplasm. A positive result is strong evidence for a prostatic tumor. A negative result, though less conclusive, is evidence for nonprostatic origin. The assay is particularly appro-priate for aspirates from metastases of unknown origin. It also can be applied to prostatic aspirates to distinguish rectal mucosal cells which can mimic microacini of well-differentiated prostatic carcinoma (see Chapter 6), or to distinguish between a primary prostatic tumor and a bladder or rectal carcinoma invading the prostate.

The current directions of immunohistochemistry in prostatic carcinoma are stud-ies of new specific antigens and of better methods to demonstrate acid phosphatase, a known antigen. An antigen discovered within the last few years is prostate-specific antigen,[36] a protein apparently specific for prostatic tissue and distinct from acid phosphatase. The sensitivity and specificity of the immunoperoxidase demonstration of prostate-specific antigen for prostatic carcinoma are similar to values for PAP—close to 100%.[2,24,29,34] Similar to the acid phosphatase reaction, very poorly dif-ferentiated carcinoma may react negatively to prostate-specific antigen.[7,34] Com-parison between prostatic acid phosphatase and prostate-specific antigen staining has shown a few tumors that are positive for prostate-specific antigen but negative for acid phosphatase.[2,7] On the other hand, some neoplasms positive for both

TABLE 7.2. Prostatic Acid Phosphatase Reactivity in Non-Prostatic Carcinomas

NAB Sites	No. Cases	Reactivity
Breast	6	2*
Lymph node metastases†	6	—
Soft tissue metastases‡	2	—
Pancreas	2	—
Lung	3	—
Thyroid	2	—

* Weak reactivity.
† Primary sites: lung (2), colon (2), esophagus (adenosquamous carcinoma) (1), ovary (1).
‡ Primary sites: lung, colon (one each).

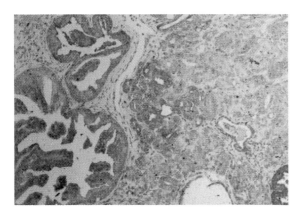

Plate 1. Well-differentiated prostatic carcinoma, histologic section. Section is stained with peroxidase antiperoxidase and hematoxylin (with no eosin). Note diffuse red cytoplasmic staining representing PAP positivity in both benign and malignant glands. Peroxidase antiperoxidase and hematoxylin. × 125.

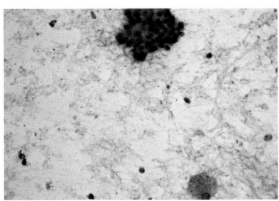

Plate 2. Benign prostatic enlargement, ABC. Note benign cell cluster with fine red cytoplasmic granules of PAP positivity, easily discernible despite extracellular background stain. Note histiocyte with coarse red cytoplasmic granules, possibly reflecting previous phagocytosis of PAP-positive material Peroxidase antiperoxidase and hematoxylin. × 300.

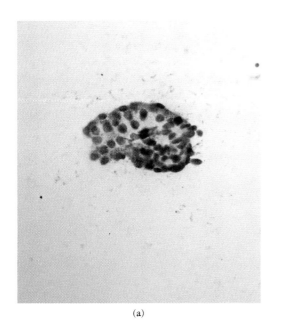

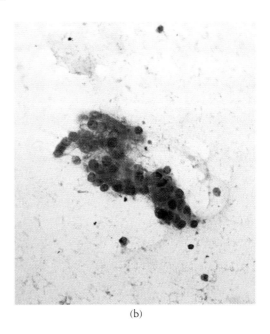

(a) (b)

Plate 3. Well-differentiated prostatic carcinoma, ABC. A. Note red cytoplasmic staining, reflecting PAP positivity only at periphery of cluster. Cytoplasm of central cells is unstained. Peroxidase antiperoxidase and hematoxylin. × 300. B. Note cytoplasmic PAP positivity diffusely throughout cell cluster. Peroxidase antiperoxidase and hematoxylin. × 300.

121

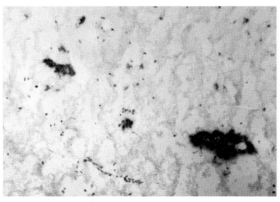

Plate 4. Moderately to poorly differentiated prostatic carcinoma, ABC. Note easily detectable PAP-positive granules under this low magnification. Peroxidase antiperoxidase and hematoxylin. ×125.

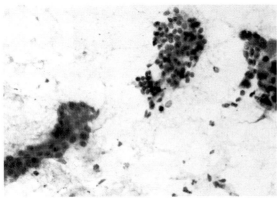

Plate 5. Well to moderately differentiated prostatic carcinoma, ABC. Note equal degree of PAP positivity in the more differentiated cell clusters (center and left) and in the less differentiated cluster (right). Peroxidase antiperoxidase and hematoxylin. ×300.

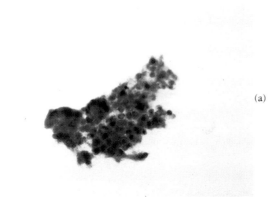

(a)

Plate 6. Prostatic carcinoma metastatic to cervical lymph node, ABC. **A**. Note diffuse cytoplasmic PAP positivity in cell group. Peroxidase antiperoxidase and hematoxylin. ×300. **B**. Note PAP positivity in cytoplasm of single cells. Peroxidase antiperoxidase and hematoxylin. ×500.

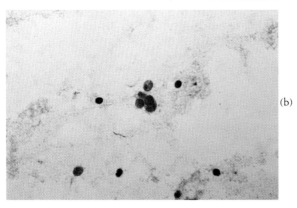

(b)

122

antigens in some areas may stain only for acid phosphatase.[2] These results suggest that some carcinomas may need examination for multiple antigens to establish the prostate as the tissue of origin.

One of the new methods for antigen detection is by monoclonal antibodies.[22,25,33] Standard antisera are polyclonal; they contain many different species of antibody reacting with different loci on the antigen or its contaminants and are obtained from repeated bleedings of animals immunized with antigen. Monoclonal antibodies are secreted by cell lines in tissue culture that have been formed from the fusion of a single antibody-producing spleen cell and a myeloma cell in culture. The fused cell takes on some of each cell's attributes: the myeloma cell imparts the ability to survive indefinitely in tissue culture; the spleen cell imparts the ability to secrete antibody specific for the antigen. Thus, there is a constant supply of each particular monoclonal antibody. The supply is unaffected by changes in an immunized animal, and, since antibodies to impurities are absent, the antiserum is highly specific for one antigenic determinant on the antigen. Monoclonal antibodies offer the promise of increased specificity and more reproducible assays. Currently, however, monoclonal antibodies for PAP are less sensitive than polyclonal antisera,[22,25,33] giving lower proportions of positive cases and often requiring frozen, rather than fixed, tissue. The combination of several different monoclonal antibodies in a "cocktail" may increase sensitivity.

Other new approaches for antigen detection include variations of the immunoperoxidase technique that have potentially greater sensitivity, such as a biotin-avidin system or a four-layer bridging technique.[25] These techniques have only recently been introduced and need to be tested extensively with clinical material.

REFERENCES

1. Abbott LB, Wenger WC, Lott JA: Acid phosphatase. In Kaplan LA, Pesce AJ: *Clinical Chemistry: Theory, Analysis, and Correlation*. St. Louis, CV Mosby, 1984, pp. 1079–1084.

2. Allhoff EP, Proppe KH, Chapman CM, Lin CW, Prout GR, Jr: Evaluation of prostate specific acid phosphatase and prostate specific antigen in identification of prostatic cancer. *J Urol* 129:315–318, 1983.

3. Bates RJ, Chapman CM, Prout GR, Jr, Lin CW: Immunohistochemical identification of prostatic acid phosphatase: correlation of tumor grade with acid phosphatase distribution. *J Urol* 127:574–580, 1982.

4. Bentz MS, Cohen C, Demers LM, Budgeon LR: Immunohistochemical acid phosphatase level and tumor grade in prostatic carcinoma. *Arch Pathol Lab Med* 106:476–480, 1982.

5. Choe BK, Pontes EJ, Rose NR, Henderson MD: Expression of human prostatic acid phosphatase in a pancreatic islet cell carcinoma. *Invest Urol* 15:312–318, 1978.

6. Choe BK, Rose NR: Prostatic acid phosphatase: a marker for human prostatic adenocarcinoma. *Methods Can Res* 19:199–232, 1982.

7. Ellis DW, Leffers S, Davies JS, Ng ABP: Multiple immunoperoxidase markers in benign hyperplasia and adenocarcinoma of the prostate. *Am J Clin Pathol* 81:279–284, 1984.

8. Esposti PL: Cytologic diagnosis of prostatic tumors with the aid of transrectal aspiration biopsy: a critical review of 1,110 cases and a report of morphologic and cytochemical studies. *Acta Cytol* 10:182–186, 1966.

9. Filmus JE, Podhajcer OL, Mareso E, Guman N, Mordoh J: Acid phosphatase in human breast cancer tissue. *Cancer* 53:301–305, 1984.

10. Fishleder A, Tubbs RR, Levin HS: An immunoperoxidase technique to aid in the differential diagnosis of prostatic carcinoma. *Cleve Clin Q* 48:331–335, 1981.

11. Foti AG, Cooper JF, Herschman H, Malvaez RR: Detection of prostatic cancer by solid-phase radioimmunoassay of serum prostatic acid phosphatase. *N Engl J Med* 297:1357–1361, 1977.

12. Gutman AB, Gutman EB: An "acid" phosphatase occurring in the serum of patients with metastasizing carcinoma of the prostate gland. *J Clin Invest* 17:473–478, 1938.

13. Jobsis AC, DeVries GP, Anholt RRH, Sanders GTB: Demonstration of the prostatic origin of metastases: an immunohistochemical method for formalin-fixed embedded tissue. *Cancer* 41:1788–1793, 1978.

14. Jobsis AC, DeVries GP, Meijer AEFH, Ploem JS: The immunohistochemical detection of prostatic acid phosphatase: its possibilities and limitations in tumour histochemistry. *Histochem J* 13:961–973, 1981.

15. Keshgegian AA, Kline TS: Immunoperoxidase demonstration of prostatic acid phosphatase in aspiration biopsy cytology. *Am J Clin Pathol* 82:586–588, 1984.

16. Lam KW, Li CY, Yam LT, Smith RS, Hacker B: Comparison of prostatic and nonprostatic acid phosphatase. *Ann NY Acad Sci* 390:1–15, 1982.

17. Li CY, Lam WKW, Yam LT: Immunohistochemical diagnosis of prostatic cancer with metastases. *Cancer* 46:706–712, 1980.

18. Lippert MC, Bensimon H, Javadpour N: Immunoperoxidase staining of acid phosphatase in human prostatic tissue. *J Urol* 128:1114–1116, 1982.

19. Mahan DE, Bruce AW, Manley PN, Franchi L: Immunohistochemical evaluation of prostatic carcinoma before and after radiotherapy. *J Urol* 124:488–491, 1980.

20. McDonald DF, Schofield BH, Geffert MA, Coleman RA: A comparative study of new substrates for the histochemical demonstration of acid phosphomonoesterase activity in tissues which secrete acid phosphatase. *J Histochem Cytochem* 28:316–322, 1980.

21. Nadji M: The potential value of immunoperoxidase techniques in diagnostic cytology. *Acta Cytol* 24:442–447, 1980.

22. Nadji M, Morales AR: Immunohistochemistry of prostatic acid phosphatase. *Ann NY Acad Sci* 390:133–141, 1982.

23. Nadji M, Tabei SZ, Castro A, Chu TM, Morales AR: Prostatic origin of tumors: an immunohistochemical study. *Am J Clin Pathol* 73:735–739, 1980.

24. Nadji M, Tabei SZ, Castro A, Chu TM, Murphy GP, Wang MC, Morales AR: Prostate-specific antigen: an immunohistologic marker for prostatic neoplasms. *Cancer* 48:1229–1232, 1981.

25. Naritoku WY, Taylor CR: A comparative study of the use of monoclonal antibodies using three different histochemical methods: an evaluation of monoclonal and polyclonal antibodies against human prostatic acid phosphatase. *J Histochem Cytochem* 30:253–260, 1982.

26. Pearse AGE: *Histochemistry, Theoretical and Applied.* vol 1, 2nd ed. Boston, Little, Brown, 1968, pp. 547–575.

27. Pontes JE: Biological markers in prostate cancer. *J Urol* 130:1037–1047, 1983.

28. Pontes JE, Rose NR, Ercole C, Pierce JM, Immunofluorescence for prostatic acid phosphatase: clinical applications. *J Urol* 126:187–189, 1981.

29. Purnell DM, Heatfield BM, Trump BF: Immunocytochemical evaluation of human prostatic carcinomas for carcinoembryonic antigen, nonspecific cross-reacting antigen, β-chorionic gonadotrophin, and prostate-specific antigen. *Cancer Res* 44:285–292, 1984.

30. Romas NA: Prostatic acid phosphatase: current concepts. *Semin Urol* 1:177–185, 1983.

31. Serrano JA, Wasserkrug HL, Serrano AA, Paul BD, Seligman AM: The histochemical demonstration of human prostatic acid phosphatase with phosphorylcholine. *Invest Urol* 15:123–136, 1977.

32. Sheehan DC, Hrapchak BB: *Theory and Practice of Histotechnology.* 2nd ed. St. Louis, CV Mosby, 1980, pp. 298–300.

33. Shevchuk MM, Romas NA, Ng PY, Tannenbaum M, Olsson CA: Acid phosphatase localization in prostatic carcinoma: a comparison of monoclonal antibody to heteroantisera. *Cancer* 52:1642–1646, 1983.

34. Stein BS, Peterson RO, Vangore S, Kendall AR: Immunoperoxidase localization of prostate-specific antigen. *Am J Surg Pathol* 6:553–557, 1982.

35. Troster M, Grignon D: Changes in immunohistochemical staining in prostatic adenocarcinoma following diethylstilbestrol therapy. *Lab Invest* (abstr) 50:60A–61A, 1984.

36. Wang MC, Valenzuela LA, Murphy GP, Chu TM: Purification of a human prostate specific antigen. *Invest Urol* 17:159–163, 1979.

37. Yam LT, Janckila AJ, Lam WKW, Li CY: Immunohistochemistry of prostatic acid phosphatase. *The Prostate* 2:97–107, 1981.

38. Yam LT, Winkler CF, Janckila AJ, Li CY, Lam KW: Prostatic cancer presenting as metastatic adenocarcinoma of unknown origin: immunodiagnosis by prostatic acid phosphatase. *Cancer* 51:283–287, 1983.

8

Application of Needle Aspiration Biopsy After Diagnosis of Cancer

INTRODUCTION

Subsequent to diagnosis of cancer of the prostate, fine-needle biopsy can supply vital data. Initially, it can be used for staging the tumor. After treatment, it can provide assessment of the gland for recurrence and of adjacent tissue and distant sites for metastases. These biopsies may be performed from visible and palpable masses in the office or in the x-ray suite under guidance by fluoroscopy, ultrasonography, or computerized tomography.

Prognosis of cancer of the prostate is directly linked to its size and spread. Curative therapy can be administered only when it is confined to the gland. Thus, for the purpose of treatment and prognosis, four stages have been designated[22]:

Stage A: Clinically inapparent cancer incidentally discovered at surgery or autopsy

This lesion, totally within the prostate, is subdivided into focal stage A1 disease and diffuse stage A2 disease. Patients with stage A disease represent about 10% of all prostate carcinomas.[20]

Stage B: Palpable carcinoma confined to the prostate

This stage, too, is divided into focal stage B1 and diffuse stage B2. Approximately 10–15% of the cases are discovered in this stage.[20]

Stage C: Tumors which have penetrated the capsule of the prostate but have not metastasized

Initial diagnosis of patients in stage C represents approximately 40% of the total.[8]

Stage D: Metastatic cancer

Stage D1 carcinoma has metastasized to the pelvic nodes, and stage D2 indicates distant metastases. Almost 40% of all patients first are diagnosed at this late stage.[20]

Clinical estimates of tumor parameters are inaccurate and invariably underestimated.[20] Needle aspiration biopsy, however, can be of aid in the assessment of the volume of the tumor and its clinical stage and, consequently, in the delineation of therapeutic options and curative potential, particularly regarding the value of radical prostatectomy. From Scandinavian data,[7] NAB has proved unprofitable for establishing diagnosis in patients without palpable nodules (stage A cancer). For diagnosis of stage B disease, however, it is invaluable, and multiple biopsies may indicate whether malignant cells are confined to a single area or dispersed throughout the gland. For identification of stage C carcinoma, seminal vesicles, corpus cavernosum, bladder, or rectum may be accurately explored by transrectal or percutaneous fine-needle biopsy. Stage D carcinoma may be diagnosed in patients with previously treated tumor or in patients who first present because of metastases (occult carcinoma).

POST-THERAPY EVALUATION OF THE PROSTATE

After therapy for carcinoma, palpation of the prostate often is inadequate for evaluation. With orchiectomy or hormonal medication, findings may be equivocal, and after irradiation a stony-hard texture is not necessarily indicative of recurrence. Schmidt et al,[19] in a study on the effects of chemotherapy for patients with advanced prostatic carcinoma, wrote that their greatest difficulty was the lack of an adequate, objective indicator of tissue response.

Subsequent to treatment, NAB from the prostate without recurrent tumor usually reveals sparse cells from the gland. Aspiration biopsy cytology is composed chiefly of squamous cells originating in metaplastic cell nests (see Chapter 3, section on

TABLE 8.1. Correlation of Clinical Results and Aspiration Biopsy Cytology—
55 Treated Patients*

Estimated Size† (cu mm) (No. Patients)	ABC		
	Carcinoma	Suspicious	Benign
Minuscule (9)	0	0	9
0.5 (12)	3	1	8
1.5 (12)	4	3	5
2.5 (7)	2	1	4
4 (9)	8	0	1
Large, firm shelf (6)	6	0	0

* (From Kline TS, Kohler FP, Kelsey DM: Aspiration biopsy cytology (ABC): its use in diagnosis of lesions of the prostate gland. *Arch Pathol Lab Med* 106:136–139, 1982.)
† Per rectum.

Squamous Metaplasia). In addition, there are histiocytes and some inflammatory cells. Aspiration biopsy cytology from recurrent carcinoma treated by hormones or orchiectomy is interpreted in the same way as the aspirate from primary carcinoma. Aspiration biopsy cytology from the irradiated prostate (6,000–7,000 rads) also may be interpreted in this manner but occasionally results in diagnostic pitfalls (see Chapter 9, section on Interpretative Traps). From examination of 55 patients following various modes of therapy, the barely palpable gland (miniscule) always correlated with benign ABC while the firm, large, shelf-like lesion invariably showed carcinoma cells. Interestingly, nodules clinically estimated from 0.5 to 2.5 cu mm in area could not be evaluated accurately by rectal examination alone.[12] (Table 8.1; Figs. 8.1–8.6).

EVALUATION OF SUPERFICIAL MASSES: SOFT TISSUE AND LYMPH NODES

Invasion of perineural lymphatics is a common finding in carcinoma of the prostate, and metastases to lymph nodes occur early. Pelvic and lumbar nodes are involved initially, followed by periaortic, mediastinal, and bronchial nodes and, lastly, by supraclavicular and cervical nodes.[6]

Percutaneous NAB is meritorious for evaluation of superficial masses.[11] Pollen[16] cited its reliability in differentiating metastases from hematomas, bladder distension, benign soft tissue masses, or lymph nodes. For these patients, puncture can be undertaken easily and successfully in the office with a 30-mm, 22-gauge disposable needle and 3–5-cc syringe (see Chapter 2, section on Superficial Soft Tissue Masses) (Fig. 8.7).

Benign lymphadenopathy may be distinguished from metastatic carcinoma with an accuracy of 95%.[13] Aspiration biopsy cytology from the hyperplastic node is cell-dense with isolated, polymorphic lymphoid elements. The predominant cell is the small lymphocyte (6–7 μm in diameter), and there also are a few large lymphocytes (8–9 μm in diameter), elongated fibroblasts, small histiocytes, neutrophils, plasma cells, and occasional macrophages. By contrast, ABC from metastatic carcinoma reveals a few or many cells alien to the lymph node; these cells are often several times larger than lymphoid cells and are frequently in dyshesive clusters. Cells from metastatic prostatic cancer may be smaller than cells from other sites, and may range in size from 8 to 13 μm diameter. They often appear in groups of 3 to 20 loosely bound cells, sometimes forming peripheral microacini. The cells have indistinct borders, irregular nuclear membranes, and enlarged, sometimes eosinophilic nucleoli (Figs. 8.8–8.10). Whenever tissue or ABC is available from a previously diagnosed primary carcinoma, it should be compared with the metastatic malignant cells for verification of the source. In addition, particularly for occult primary sites, the tumor cells may be subjected to the immunoperoxidase technique for the presence of prostatic acid phosphatase (see Chapter 7). Negative results, of course, do not completely exclude primary carcinoma of the prostate.

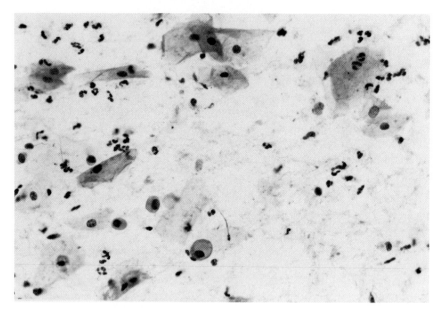

Fig. 8.1. Hormone-treated prostate, (0.5 cu mm) without recurrence, ABC. Note mature squamous, and inflammatory cells. Papanicolaou preparation. ×300.

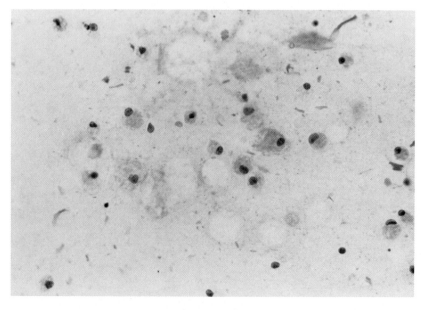

Fig. 8.2. Orchiectomy and radiation-treated prostate (miniscule) without recurrence, ABC. Note many histiocytes. Papanicolaou preparation. ×300.

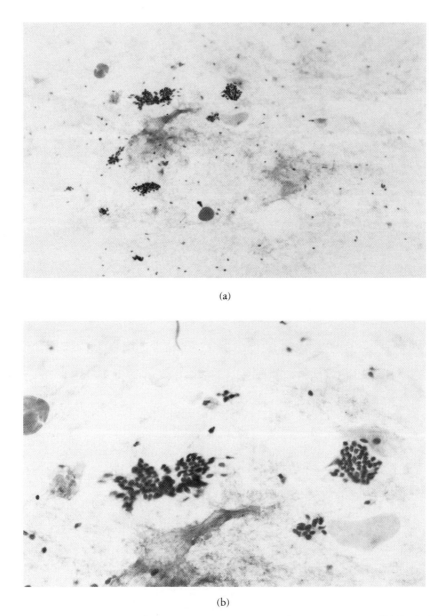

(a)

(b)

Fig. 8.3. Orchiectomy-treated prostate (1.5 cu mm) without recurrence, ABC. **A**. Note moderate cellularity. Papanicolaou preparation. × 30. **B**. Higher-magnification view. Note cohesive, polarized cell clusters. Papanicolaou preparation. × 125.

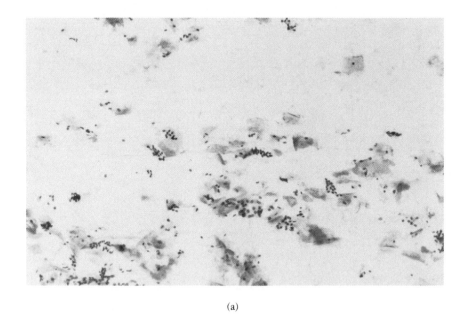

(a)

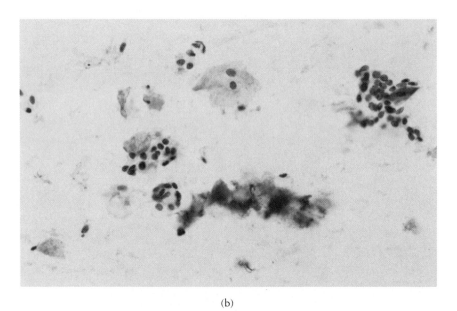

(b)

Fig. 8.4. Hormone-treated prostate (2.5 cu mm) with recurrent well-differentiated carcinoma. **A**. ABC. Note cell-rich specimen with dyshesive cells. Papanicolaou preparation. ×125. **B**. ABC. Note dyshesive cells, some forming microacini. Papanicolaou preparation. ×300.

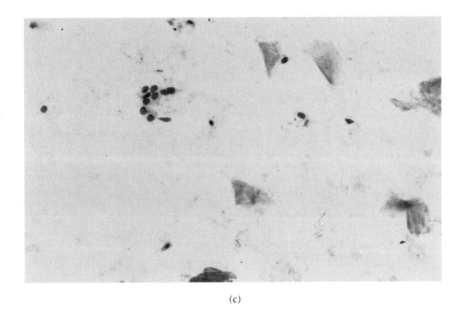

(c)

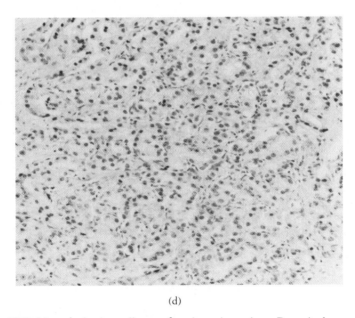

(d)

Fig. 8.4. C ABC. Note dyshesive cells, one forming microacinus. Papanicolaou preparation. × 300. **D.** Histologic section, original carcinoma. Hematoxylin and eosin preparation. × 125.

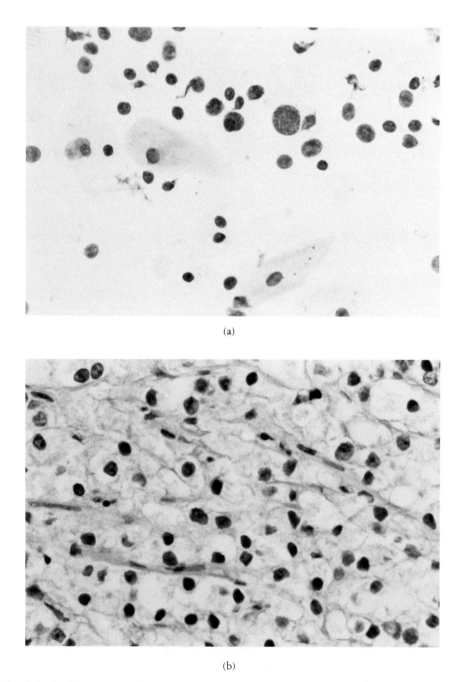

(a)

(b)

Fig. 8.5. Orchiectomy and hormone-treated prostate (0.5 cu mm) with recurrent poorly differentiated carcinoma. **A.** ABC. Note bizarre naked nuclei. Papanicolaou preparation. × 500. **B.** Histologic section, original carcinoma. Hematoxylin and eosin preparation. × 300.

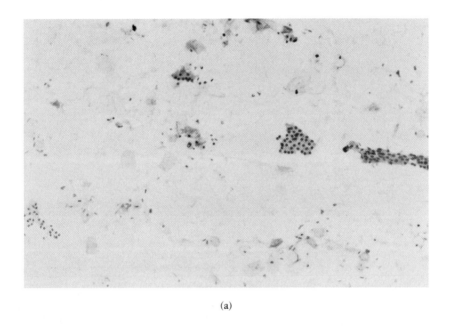

(a)

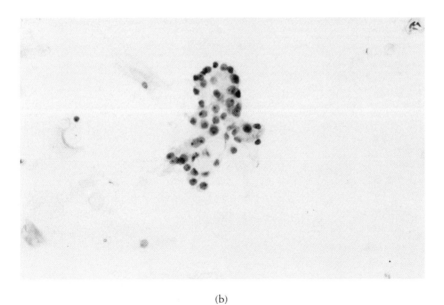

(b)

Fig. 8.6. Radiation-treated prostate (0.5 cu mm) with recurrent moderately differentiated carcinoma, ABC. **A.** Note moderate cellularity. Papanicolaou preparation. ×125. **B.** Note dyshesive group. Papanicolaou preparation. ×300.

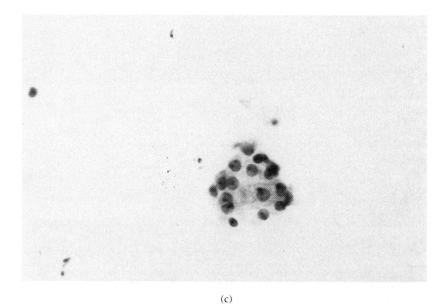

(c)

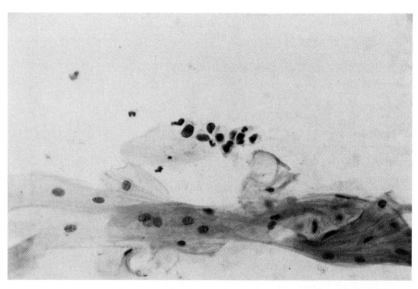

(d)

Fig. 8.6. C. Note dyshesive groups with macronucleoli. Papanicolaou preparation. ×300. **D.** Note small tumor cells with anisonucleosis and irregular nuclei. Papanicolaou preparation. ×500.

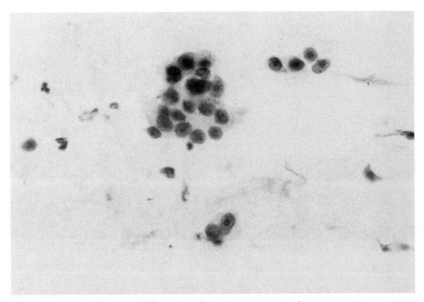

Fig. 8.7. Stage C, moderately differentiated carcinoma, extending to perineum; NAB, perineal nodule. Note dyshesive cell clusters with macronucleoli. Papanicolaou preparation. ×500.

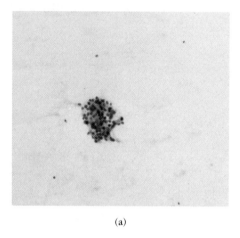

(a)

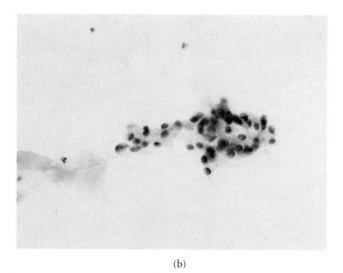

(b)

Fig. 8.8. Stage D, moderately to poorly differentiated carcinoma; NAB, cervical lymph node (see also Plate 7.6). A. Note alien cell cluster. Papanicolaou preparation. ×125. B. Note dyshesive group. Papanicolaou preparation. ×300.

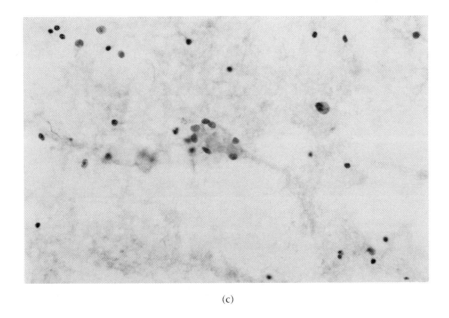

(c)

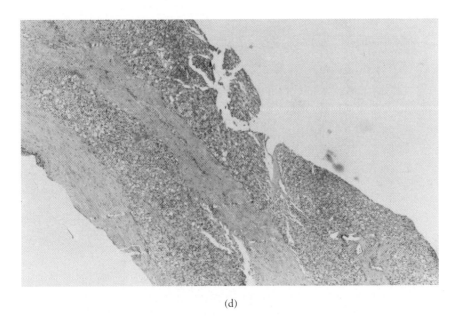

(d)

Fig. 8.8. C. Note alien cells amid lymphocytes. Papanicolaou preparation. ×300. **D**. Histologic section, original prostatic biopsy. Hematoxylin and eosin preparation. ×30.

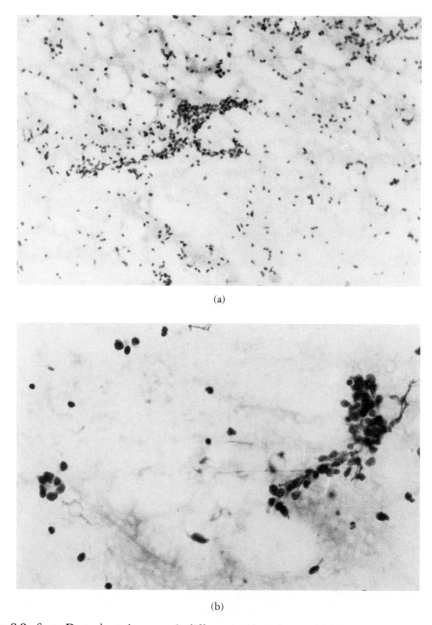

(a)

(b)

Fig. 8.9. Stage D, moderately to poorly differentiated carcinoma; NAB, cervical lymph node. **A.** Note cell-dense specimen. Papanicolaou preparation. ×125. **B.** Note alien cells. Papanicolaou preparation. ×300.

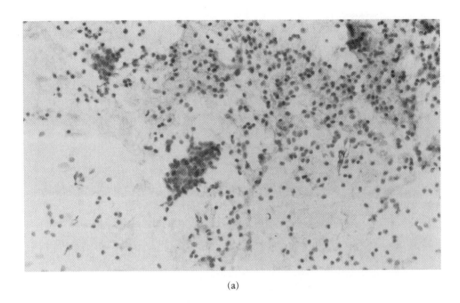

(a)

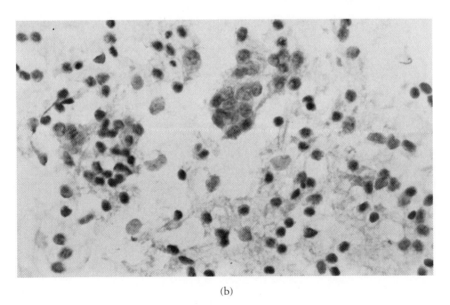

(b)

Fig. 8.10. Stage D, poorly differentiated carcinoma; NAB, peripancreatic region. **A.** Note cell-dense specimen. Papanicolaou preparation. ×125. **B.** Note dyshesive, often isolated cells. Papanicolaou preparation. ×500.

EVALUATION OF DEEP MASSES

The earliest metastases from carcinoma of the prostate are to regional lymph nodes. Node metastases were found in 93% of a series of patients graded as 8–10 by Gleason's nomenclature.[14] In an autopsy study of 104 men with cancer of the prostate, Elkin and Mueller[6] discovered osseous metastases in 65%, lung involvement (sometimes only microscopic foci) in 38%, and liver metastases in 22%. Although spread is primarily through lymphatic channels, tumor emboli also may disseminate by hematogenous routes, in part through epidural veins (Batson's plexus), and lodge in the brain.[18] Castaldo et al[1] reported intracranial metastases in 4.2% of 189 patients with stage C or D cancer. Radiographic guidance for fine-needle biopsy provides an avenue of diagnosis for all these sites of metastases.[11]

Evaluation of lymph nodes by lymphangiography in combination with aspiration biopsy has been rewarding. Efremidis et al,[5] Prando et al,[17] and Göthlin and Macintosh[9] successfully used NAB with biplane fluoroscopy to diagnose lymphangiographically suspicious nodes, and Macintosh et al[15] confirmed its effectiveness in nodes from 0.2 to 1.0 cm in diameter. Wajsman et al[21] canceled "staging" lymphadenectomy for five patients with "localized" carcinoma because of the discovery of tumor cells in the ABC from equivocal nodes.

The usefulness of radiographically directed percutaneous NAB for assessment of possible hepatic metastases is illustrated by this case:

> A 75-year-old man, treated for prostatic carcinoma, had a subsequent liver scan, interpreted as a probable metastasis. Needle aspiration biopsy, performed with computerized tomographic guidance, removed 5.0 cc of viscid, creamy fluid composed only of necrotic neutrophils. The benign abscess was drained.

Aspiration biopsy cytology can provide similar data from the lung and brain.[11]

Sites of metastases to bone, in order of decreasing frequency, are ilium, pubisischium, lumbosacral and thoracic spines, ribs, femur, and sternum.[20] Not rarely, occult prostatic cancer is discovered because of bone pain or high serum acid phosphatase, although acid phosphatase is elevated in only about 39% of the patients with bone metastases.[3] Metastatic tumor has been recovered in these patients by selective or blind bone biopsy. In the latter group, positivity proved highest in patients with elevated acid phosphatase.[3] Bone samples from all sites can be taken by aspiration biopsy in the office or under fluoroscopic guidance (see Chapter 2, section on Bone). Aspiration biopsy cytology from regions of metastatic carcinoma is diagnosed by the presence of cells alien to marrow elements (Fig. 8.11). From 379 fine needle bone biopsies, DeSantos and Zornoza[4] correctly diagnosed 78%, and reported that it was a safe and reliable method.

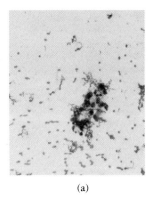

(a)

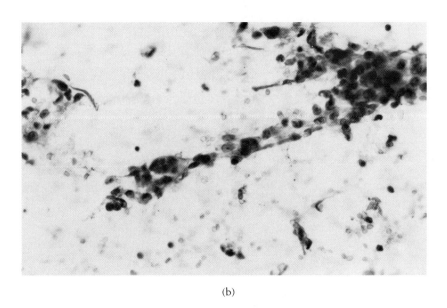

(b)

Fig. 8.11. Occult prostatic carcinoma, iliac crest. **A**. ABC, iliac crest. Note alien cells. Papanicolaou preparation. × 125. **B**. ABC, iliac crest. Note dyshesive cell clusters. Papanicolaou preparation. × 300.

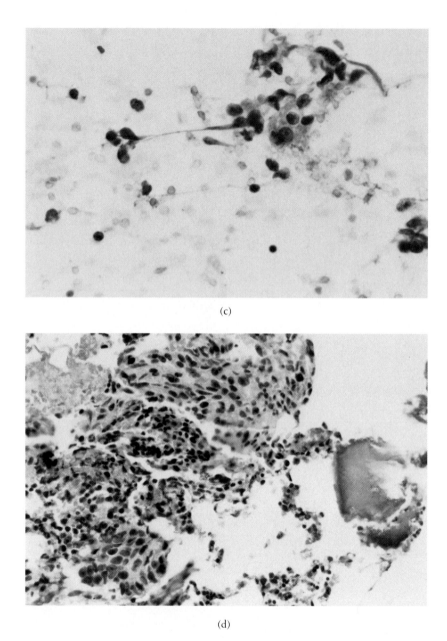

(c)

(d)

Fig. 8.11. C. ABC, iliac crest. Note cells with anisonucleosis and macronucleoli. Papanicolaou preparation. ×500. **D.** Histologic section, bone marrow. Hematoxylin and eosin preparation. ×125.

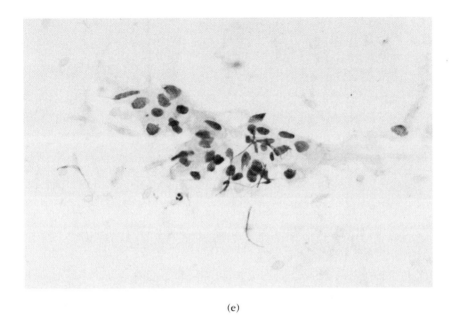

(e)

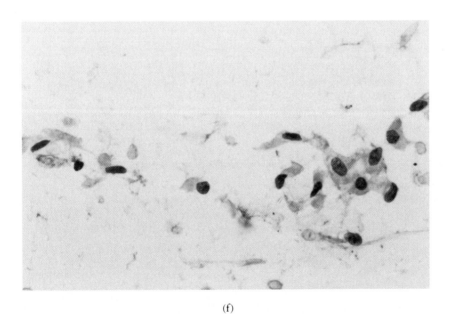

(f)

Fig. 8.11. E., F. Prostate with altered consistency, ABC. Note dyshesive tumor cells. Papanicolaou preparations. ×300, ×500.

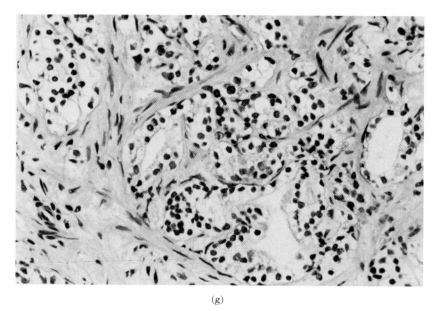

(g)

Fig. 8.11. G. Histologic section, prostatic carcinoma. Hematoxylin and eosin preparation. ×300.

A CLINICIAN'S VIEW

F. Peter Kohler

Malignant prostatic lesions, once diagnosed and treated, are especially appropriate for fine needle aspiration biopsy during follow-up examinations. It is a common experience that the mass of prostatic carcinoma diminishes within 3 months after institution of definitive therapy. It is also common experience that only a portion of these lesions actually have reverted to benignity. At this time, NAB on an outpatient basis is of great value. A clinical instance will serve as demonstration:

> *A 72-year-old man had a moderately differentiated stage C carcinoma of the prostate. Within 6 months of bilateral orchiectomy, the gland shrank from the size of a large walnut to that of a cherry. Bone scans were negative, and acid phosphatase remained normal. Two years later, the gland enlarged, and NAB again showed moderately differentiated tumor, although bone scans were negative and acid phosphatase remained normal. The patient then received cobalt therapy, 6,400 rads. Five years after discovery, the gland had diminished to the size of a lima bean but NAB again revealed carcinoma, this time poorly differentiated. Although the lesion is obviously active, it has remained localized.*

This case illustrates the way a patient can be followed with ease at any time by outpatient needle aspiration biopsies. This case also illustrates the dilemma of the significance of positive biopsies after cobalt therapy. Some argue that a positive biopsy means that the cobalt treatment was a failure. Radiotherapists, on the other hand, claim that although the cells may appear malignant, they have lost their biological potential, trapped in a fibrous envelope and unable to pass beyond this barrier. A positive biopsy in a patient with an enlarging tumor mass is obviously ominous. We believe that the patient with a positive biopsy and a tumor of static size should be observed with vigilance. We treat these lesions by whatever therapeutic mode is appropriate, because their potential biological status is essentially unknown. Herr and Whitmore[10] consider that core-biopsy specimens taken at intervals after completion of treatment is the only method for "objective" assessment of local effects of radiotherapy. We have concluded that in this endeavor, NAB of the prostate is the solution.

Another area of concern in the literature is the predictability of pelvic lymph node metastases based on the histologic grade of the carcinoma obtained by core-needle biopsy. Catalone et al.[2] are of the opinion that core-needle biopsy is associated with a significant error in grading, and question whether the correlation between tumor grade and lymph node metastases is sufficiently accurate in stage B disease to allow decisions for future therapy. In opposition, Zincke et al[23] believe that patients with a grade 1 or grade 2 tumor, and a well- to moderately differentiated carcinoma no greater than 2.0 cm in diameter, require no pelvic lymphadenectomy for diagnostic or therapeutic reasons. It is our opinion that grading by ABC is at least as accurate as by core biopsy, and that it is possible to base decision for lymphadenectomy on this approach.

Two cases illustrate the special application of NAB following radical perineal prostatectomy:

> A 65 year-old man, found to have a stage A, poorly differentiated carcinoma, had a radical perineal prostatectomy. Follow-up studies were normal for 5 years. Then a pea-size ridge became palpable at the suture line in the area of the membranous urethra. Aspiration biopsy cytology showed malignant cells, and a bilateral orchiectomy was performed. Three months later, no prostatic tissue was palpable in the area.

> A 58-year-old man had a radical perineal prostatectomy for poorly differentiated stage B carcinoma. Bone scans and acid phosphatase remained normal for 7 years until a match-size ridge between vesical neck and membranous urethra became palpable. Aspiration biopsy cytology showed recurrent carcinoma. He also developed a metastasis in the body of the sixth thoracic vertebra. Bilateral orchiectomy was performed, and the ridge of tissue disappeared.

Core-needle biopsies in these patients would have been hazardous because of possible fistula formation; in addition, crush artifacts may have precluded definitive histologic diagnosis.

In urologic disease, the prostate is the obvious tissue available for NAB, but the clinician always must be alert to the possible use of this technique in other anatomic areas. Suspicious lesions of the spermatic cord and testis lend themselves particularly well to NAB. Needle aspiration biopsy of the testis is frowned upon as a routine procedure because it is argued that the needle tract serves as a source of tumor contamination and a field for future metastases to the spermatic fasciae and the scrotal skin. No evidence in the literature, however, supports this contention. We, therefore, have resorted to fine-needle aspiration of testicular masses which are of a suspicious nature:

> A 58-year-old physician noticed a gradual increase in size of his left testis and, simultaneously, left inguinal lymphadenopathy and chills and fever. A urologist interpreted the findings as an infectious process and treated him with antibiotics. Four months later, the

inguinal nodes were the same size but firmer, and the testis, though less tender, was hard throughout. Despite a normal radionucleotide scan of the testis, the patient was advised to have exploratory scrotal surgery which he refused and sought another opinion. On examination, there were two lima-bean-size firm, left inguinal lymph nodes. The left testis was stony-hard but normal in shape and size. The left epididymis was still tender and about twice normal size. Needle aspiration biopsy of the testis was reported as benign, but ABC from the lymph nodes suggested lymphoma. The nodes were surgically removed and showed histiocytic lymphoma, and a lymphangiogram showed involvement of the left external and common iliac chain with extension to the pariaortic level at the fourth lumbar vertebra. After treatment with chemotherapy, the left testis gradually returned to normal elasticity, and the epididymis regressed to normal size.

(See Fig. 8.12) This patient was diagnosed and treated without major surgery, strictly on an ambulatory basis because of the use of NAB.

In the field of urology, NAB has been exceedingly helpful. From an economic point of view, it allows diagnosis and treatment on an outpatient basis with a minimum of discomfort and complications for the patient. From a clinical point of view, this method of diagnosis is as accurate, in our experience, as any other biopsy method. It is much less destructive of tissue than the True-cut or Vim-Silverman needles. The fine needle can be guided to the suspicious area with ease and is less likely to cause tumor spread in the periprostatic tissues. Needle aspiration biopsy will be welcomed by all clinicians once they are familiar with the procedure and have the cooperative support from the pathologist.

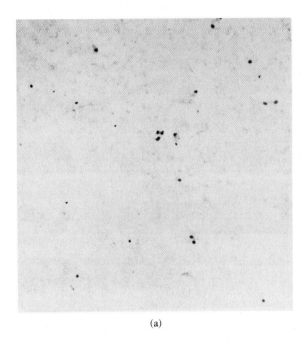

(a)

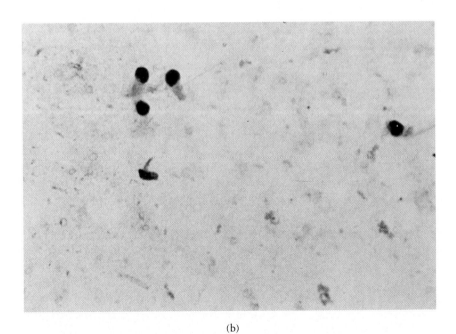

(b)

Fig. 8.12. Inguinal lymphadenopathy and testicular firmness. **A.** Testis, ABC. Note modest cellularity. Papanicolaou preparation. ×125. **B.** Testis, ABC. Note isolated, slender Sertoli cells. Papanicolaou preparation. ×500.

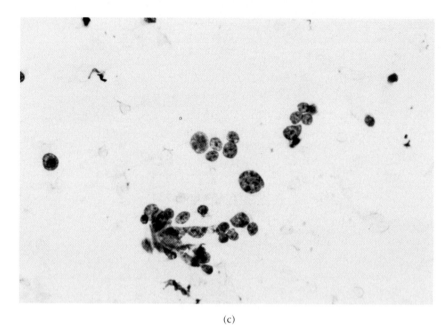

(c)

Fig. 8.12. C. Inguinal lymph node, histiocytic lymphoma, ABC. Note monomorphic lymphoid cells with anisonucleosis and macronucleoli. Papanicolaou preparation. × 500.

REFERENCES

1. Castaldo JE, Bernat JL, Meier FA, Schned AR: Intracranial metastases due to prostatic carcinoma. *Cancer* 52:1739–1747, 1983.

2. Catalone WJ, Stein AJ, Fair WR: Grading errors in prostatic needle biopsies; relation to the accuracy of tumor grade in predicting pelvic lymph node metastases. *J Urol* 127:919–922, 1982.

3. Chua DT, Ackermann W, Veenema RJ: Bone marrow biopsy in patients with carcinoma of the prostate. *J Urol* 102:602–609, 1969.

4. DeSantos LA, Zornoza J: Bone and soft tissue. In Zornoza J: *Percutaneous Needle Biopsy*. Baltimore, Williams & Wilkins, 1981, pp. 141–178.

5. Efremidis SC, Pagliarulo A, Dan SJ, Weber HN, Dillon RN, Nieburgs H, Mitty HA: Post-lymphangiography fine needle aspiration lymph node biopsy in staging carcinoma of the prostate: preliminary report. *J Urol* 122:495–497, 1979.

6. Elkin M, Mueller HP: Metastases from cancer of the prostate; autopsy and roentgenological findings. *Cancer* 7:1246–1248, 1954.

7. Esposti PL: Aspiration biopsy and cytological evaluation for primary diagnosis and follow-up. In Jacobi GH, Hohenfellner R: *Prostate Cancer. International Perspectives in Urology*, vol 3. Baltimore, Williams and Wilkins, 1982, pp. 71–92.

8. Flocks RH: Clinical cancer of the prostate; a study of 4,000 cases. *JAMA* 193:559–562, 1965.

9. Göthlin JH, Macintosh PK: Interventional radiology in the assessment of the retroper-

itoneal lymph nodes. In Macintosh PK, Thomson KR: Symposium on Interventional Radiology. *Radiol Clin N Am* 27:461–475, 1979.

10. Herr HW, Whitmore WF, Jr: Significance of prostatic biopsies after radiation therapy for carcinoma of the prostate. *The Prostate* 3:339–350, 1982.

11. Kline TS: *Handbook of Fine Needle Aspiration Biopsy Cytology.* St. Louis, CV Mosby, 1981.

12. Kline TS, Kohler FP, Kelsey DM: Aspiration biopsy cytology (ABC); its use in diagnosis of lesions of the prostate gland. *Arch Pathol Lab Med* 106:136–139, 1982.

13. Kline TS, Kannan V, Kline IK: Lymphadenopathy and ABC (aspiration biopsy cytology); review of 376 superficial nodes. *Cancer* 54:1076–1081, 1984.

14. Kramer SA, Spahr J, Brendler CB, Glenn JF, Paulson DF: Experience with Gleason's histopathologic grading in prostatic cancer. *J Urol* 124:223–225, 1980.

15. Macintosh PK, Thomson KR, Barbaric ZL: Percutaneous transperitoneal lymph-node biopsy as a means of improving lymphographic diagnosis. *Radiology* 131:647–649, 1979.

16. Pollen JJ, Schmidt JD: Diagnostic fine needle aspiration of soft tissue metastases from cancer of the prostate. *J Urol* 121:59–61, 1979.

17. Prando A, Wallace S, Von Eschenbach AC, Jing B, Rosengren J, Hussey DH: Lymphangiography in staging of carcinoma of the prostate. *Radiology* 131:641–645, 1979.

18. Saphir O: *A Text on Systemic Pathology.* New York, Grune & Stratton, 1958, pp. 736–753.

19. Schmidt, JD, Johnson DE, Scott WW, Gibbons RP, Prout GR, Murphy GP: Chemotherapy of advanced prostatic cancer; evaluation of response parameters. *Urology* 7:602–610, 1976.

20. Stamey TA: Cancer of the prostate; an analysis of some important contributions and dilemmas. *Monogr Urol* 4:68–92, 1983.

21. Wajsman Z, Gamarra M, Park JJ, Beckley S, Pontas JE: Transabdominal fine needle aspiration of retroperitoneal lymph nodes in staging of genitourinary tract cancer; correlation with lymphography and lymph node dissection findings. *J Urol* 128:1238–1240, 1982.

22. Whitmore WF: The rationale and results of ablative surgery for prostatic cancer. *Cancer* 16:1119–1132, 1963.

23. Zincke H, Farrow GM, Myers RP, Benson RC Jr, Furlow WL, Utz DC: Relationship between grade and stage of adenocarcinoma of the prostate and regional pelvic lymph node metastases. *J Urol* 128:498–501, 1982.

9

Diagnostic Problems

HISTOLOGIC CONFIRMATION OF PROSTATIC CARCINOMA

Verification of the ABC, positive for carcinoma, by corresponding tissue biopsy from the prostate is not always possible. By contrast to the rigid varieties of biopsy tools, the flexible, thin needle can be guided directly into a small malignant nodule or focal latent carcinoma. Transurethral resection, which samples periurethral tissue, is the least accurate method for demonstrating the neoplasm. Core biopsy also may miss the lesion: in a study of 139 patients with carcinoma,[16] the presence of the tumor sometimes only could be corroborated in the second, third, or even fourth transperineal biopsy. With suprapubic prostatectomy, the significant outer rim adjacent to the rectum may not be removed. The seldom-performed total prostatectomy is the single definitive surgical procedure for confirmation of the carcinoma.

Our own cases and those from other studies illustrate the problem of histologic confirmation. Nine of our 158 patients with carcinoma by needle aspiration biopsy required at least two biopsies prior to histologic verification,[21] and two additional cases are presented in the Clinical Prologue and Figures 9.1 and 9.2. Ward[35] had the same dilemma in 12 patients, and both he and Andersson et al[3] suggested that NAB and core biopsy should be used to complement each other. Ekman et al[10] described seven patients with positive ABC and benign or inconclusive histology, with six carcinomas documented by repeated biopsy. Ackermann and Müller,[1] with simultaneous transperineal core biopsy and NAB, ultimately confirmed the carcinoma histologically in 11 of 14 patients with malignant cells. Faul and Schmiedt[12] in a similar study, were unable to verify 23 of 254 carcinomas in the initial histologic biopsy. Of Lin and co-workers'[26] 47 patients, interpreted as having carcinoma by ABC and subsequent benign transurethral resections, 24 developed clinical, laboratory, or radiographic evidence of carcinoma, 4 showed carcinoma on repeated histologic biopsy, and 5 more had additional positive aspiration biopsies.

Thus, carcinoma, diagnosed from ABC by an experienced cytopathologist and with concomitant benign tissue sections, must be considered histologically unconfirmed rather than seemingly erroneous. All diagnoses must be evaluated in light of diagnostic pitfalls (see below).

153

DYSPLASIA

Pathology

The term "dysplasia" (basal cell hyperplasia, atypical hyperplasia, adenosis) in reference to the prostate, seldom is mentioned in the American literature. Koss,[23] in fact, has explained "dysplasia" as "not a diagnosis but an excuse to define a lesion of uncertain prognosis," a statement which certainly can be applied to the following discussion. There are few studies of its histology, significance, and prognosis. Even its existence is questioned, and Lewis[25] wrote, "there is apparently no well-recognized pre-cancerous lesion of the prostate. . . . Any new growth of tissue exhibited by new formation of acini in the posterior lamella or true prostate must be considered malignant." This concept from 1950 still prevails, and the current status of dysplasia may be compared with that of the cervix prior to the cellular studies of Papanicolaou. The time has now arrived to define the lesion and study single glands and individual cells with NAB. We can do long-term studies by ABC of men with these abnormalities in the same manner that women with dysplasia are followed by exfoliative cytology.

Reports from the brief literature deal mainly with changes in columnar and transitional epithelium adjacent to carcinoma, and even more rarely with atypical stromal hyperplasia.[4] Harbitz and Haugen[14] found small, multifocal, atypical glandular proliferations without invasion in a few prostates at autopsy. McNeal,[27] who has been involved with this lesion for more than 20 years, initially graded dysplasia according to intraductal cellular alterations. McNeal regarded proliferation of ductal cells with nuclear crowding leading to the protrusion of cell tufts into the lumen, as minimal dysplasia; according to him, moderate dysplasia included increased crowding and clumped chromatin; while nuclear pleomorphism, prominent nucleoli, and intraductal cribriform-pattern growths constituted carcinoma in situ. Later, McNeal et al[29] associated dysplasia with atypical adenomatous hyperplasia, a focal proliferation of rounded glands with irregular budding but cytologically benign cells. In his first study, McNeal[27] observed that the cellular abnormalities coexisted with 23% of 69 carcinomas and in a second study,[28] he found that these abnormalities coexisted with 58% of 45 carcinomas, and, in addition, with 26% of 78 benign lesions. In a current series of 200 autopsy-obtained, serially blocked prostates, half with carcinoma, McNeal et al noted both types of dysplasia associated with 90% of the carcinomas but with fewer than 30% of their benign cases.[29]

The biologic potential of dysplasia remains obscure. Most investigators consider it a premalignant lesion because of the frequency of coexisting carcinoma.[7,15,17,18,32,34] Rare prospective studies provide no conclusive results: Miller and Seljelid[30] defined dysplasia as a circumscribed group of acini filled with tightly packed cells with pleomorphic nuclei. In their prospective study subsequent to suprapubic prostatectomy, within 3 years 10 of 100 patients with "dysplasia" died of cancer (although histologic review suggested initial carcinoma in 5), compared with 31% of 39 patients with stage A or stage B carcinoma, and mortality rose by an additional 6% after 7 years in the cancer group alone. Miller and Seljelid summed up their uncertainties thus: "Whether it is a pre-malignant lesion or a lesion without oncological significance . . . is not clear."

Morphologic demarcation between dysplasia and well-differentiated adenocarcinoma is indistinct. Brawn[6] wrote: "The decision whether atypical glands represent adenosis (dysplasia) or adenocarcinoma often depends solely on the personal judgment of the surgical pathologist. There are no absolute histologic criteria to separate these two entities." He retrospectively reviewed 2,842 prostate specimens for definition and prognostication.[5] Histologic criteria were based on atypical but circumscribed proliferations of glands composed of cells with pleomorphic nuclei with nucleoli. Mild and moderate dysplasia were differentiated by the size of well-circumscribed nodules, while in severe dysplasia they were only partially circumscribed. Within 8 years, carcinoma developed in 6% of 108 patients with dysplasia, by contrast to the control group which had an incidence of 3%. Brawn[6] concluded: "When the diagnosis is not clear, the wisest policy is to render a benign diagnosis coupled with close clinical follow-up and rebiopsy as needed."

We diagnose dysplasia by circumscribed foci of crowded small glands lined by relatively uniform cells or by a few somewhat isolated, irregularly shaped glands lined by pleomorphic cells with irregular nuclei and macronucleoli. Some of these lesions we formerly diagnosed as latent (incidental) carcinoma. Currently, these patients are reexamined periodically by NAB and, when indicated, by core biopsy. Cases One and Two from the Clinical Prologue and Figures 9.1 and 9.2 illustrate the problems associated with interpretation of selective biopsies. There is no question that this lesion needs further elucidation with histologic sections and, importantly, ABC.

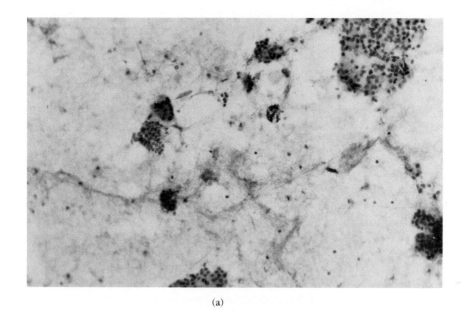

(a)

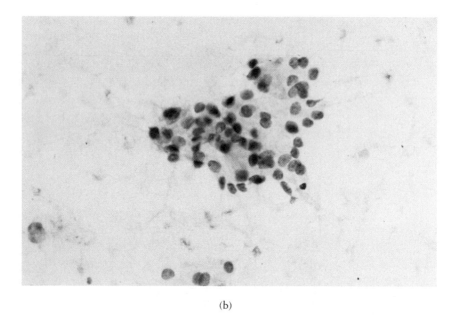

(b)

Fig. 9.1. Case One, Clinical Prologue, well-differentiated carcinoma. **A**. ABC. Note cellularity. Papanicolaou preparation. ×125. **B**. First NAB: Note dyshesive cluster with pseudoacinar formation. Papanicolaou preparation. ×300.

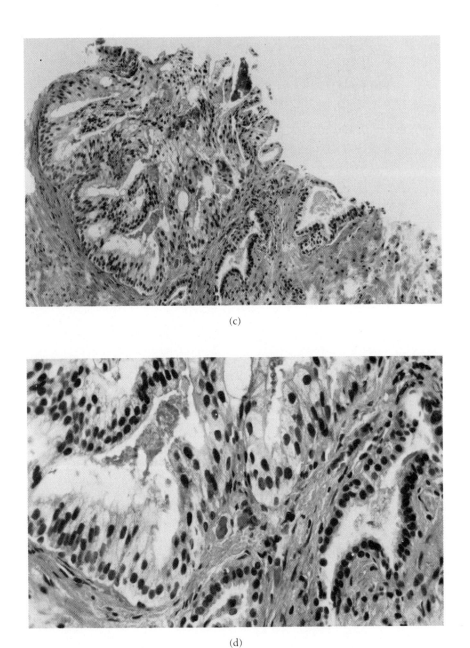

(c)

(d)

Fig. 9.1. C. Core biopsy: dysplasia. Note circumscribed collection of glands. Hematoxylin and eosin preparation. ×125. **D.** Core biopsy: dysplasia. Note cellular crowding and slight nuclear pleomorphism. Hematoxylin and eosin preparation. ×300.

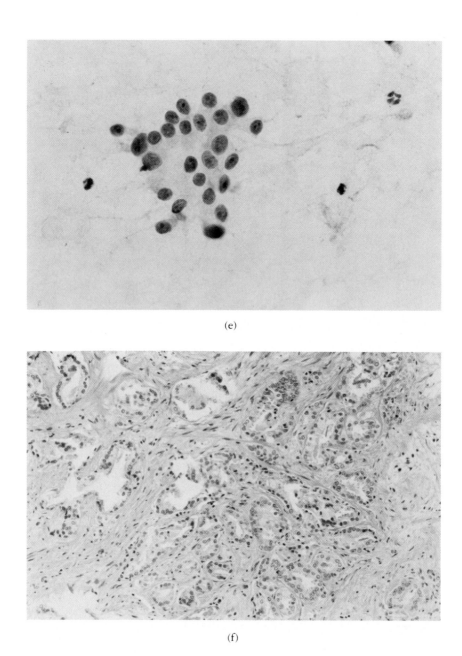

(e)

(f)

Fig. 9.1. E. Second NAB. Note small dyshesive cell cluster with anisonucleosis and macronucleoli. Papanicolaou preparation. ×500. **F.** Histologic section, open perineal biopsy: Note well-differentiated carcinoma. Hematoxylin and eosin preparation. ×125.

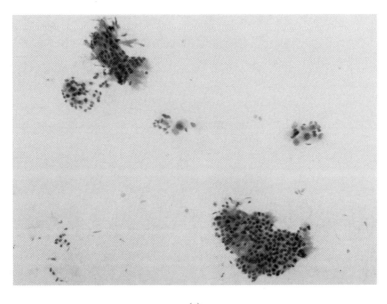

(a)

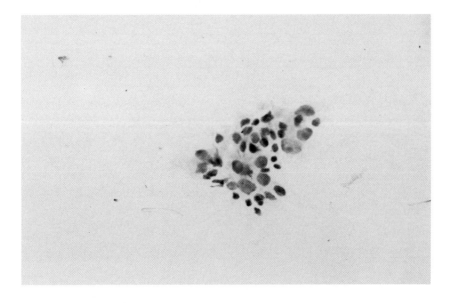

(b)

Fig. 9.2. Case Two, Clinical Prologue, moderately-differentiated carcinoma. **A**. ABC. Note cellularity and dyshesive cell groups. Papanicolaou preparation. × 125. **B**. ABC. Note dyshesive small cell group displaying anisonucleosis, nuclear membrane irregularity, macronucleoli, and indistinct cytoplasm. Papanicolaou preparation. × 300.

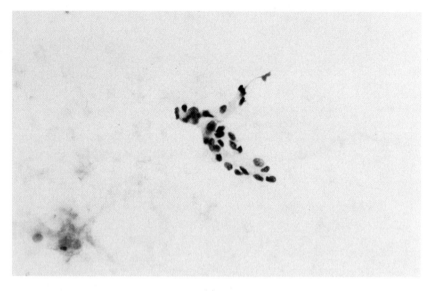

(c)

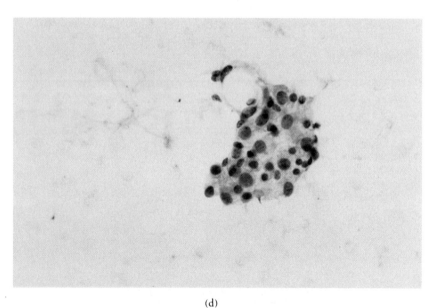

(d)

Fig. 9.2. C., D. ABC. Note dyshesive small cell groups displaying anisonucleosis, nuclear membrane irregularity, macronucleoli, and indistinct cytoplasm. Papanicolaou preparations. ×300.

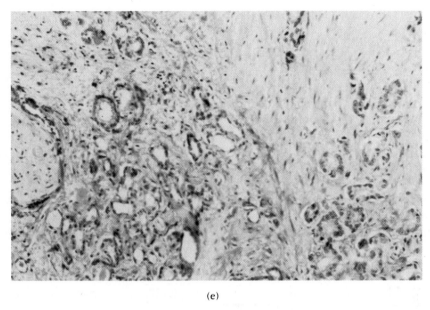

(e)

Fig. 9.2. E. Histologic section, open perineal biopsy. Note moderately differentiated adenocarcinoma, only in this third histologic biopsy. Hematoxylin and eosin preparation. × 125.

Aspiration Biopsy Cytology

Aspirates from this confusing pathologic entity reflect similar confusion. Two or three major and/or minor criteria of malignancy may be seen focally, and the pattern initially appears almost consistent with well-differentiated carcinoma. However, the examiner minutely rescreens in vain for conclusive alterations that will shift diagnosis from the suspicious into the malignant category. Cellularity may be enhanced, and rare groups may show peripheral dyshesion. There may be anisonucleosis and nuclear prominence in a few cohesive clusters, but no nuclear membrane irregularity. Cell groups may show partial loss of polarity with or without nuclear crowding, and, occasionally, there may be microacini but with minimum or no anisonucleosis (Figs. 9.1–9.6).

DeGaetani and Trentini[8] studied the ABC from 31 men with the histologic pattern of dysplasia (small, crowded acini lined by atypical cells with macronucleoli) associated with 28% of their cases of benign glandular enlargement. Aspiration biopsy cytology revealed irregular cell clumps with indistinct cell borders, rounded nuclei with finely granular chromatin, and a few small nucleoli. Kelami and Kirstaedter[19] noted similar cells with anisonucleosis. Nienhaus,[31] correlating ABC with the histologic pattern of cribriform glands and dilated glands with pseudopapillary clusters, described loss of polarity in cells with increased nuclear/cytoplasmic ratios and smooth nuclear contours.

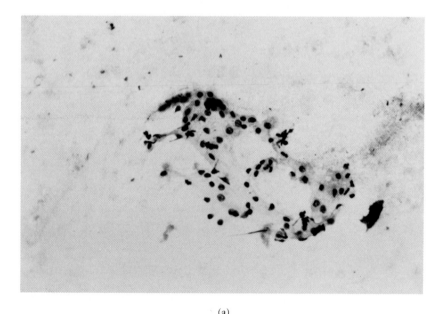

(a)

Fig. 9.3. "Suspicious" ABC followed by single benign core biopsy. **A.** Note group with loss of polarity and scalloped peripheral margins. Papanicolaou preparation. ×300.

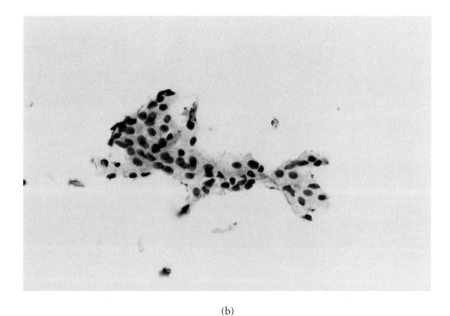

(b)

Fig. 9.3. B. Note dyshesive group with pseudoglandular formation, indistinct cell borders, and anisonucleosis. Papanicolaou preparation. × 300.

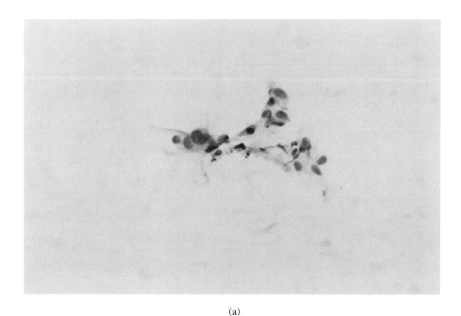

(a)

Fig. 9.4. "Suspicious" ABC followed by single benign core biopsy. **A.** Note small dyshesive group with anisonucleosis. Papanicolaou preparation. × 300.

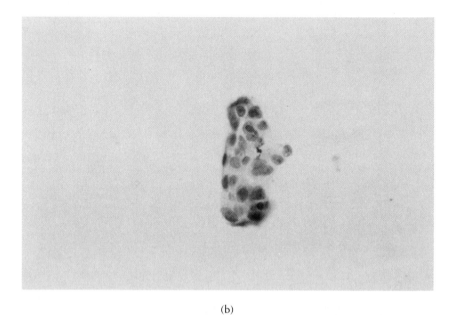

(b)

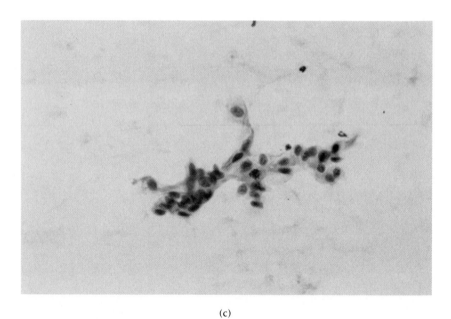

(c)

Fig. 9.4. B. Note small group with macronucleoli. Papanicolaou preparation. × 300. **C.** Note dyshesive group with indistinct cell borders and mitotic figure. Papanicolaou preparation. × 300.

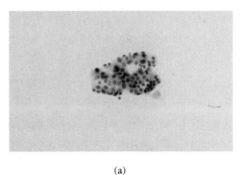

(a)

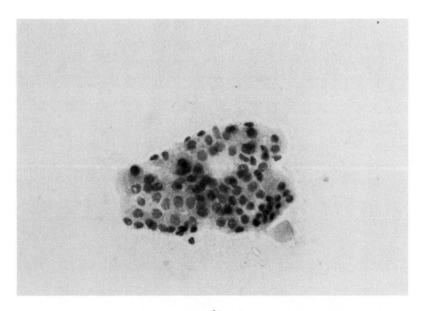

(b)

Fig. 9.5. Dysplasia. **A.** ABC. Note cell-poor specimen and cell cluster with loss of polarity. Papanicolaou preparation. × 125. **B.** ABC, higher-magnification view. Note anisonucleosis. Papanicolaou preparation. × 300.

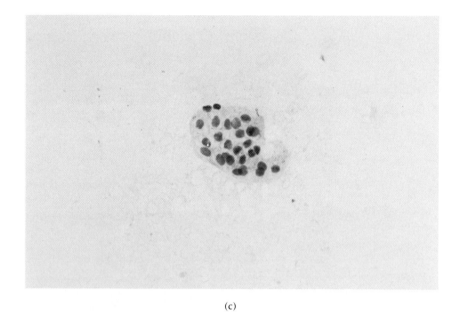

(c)

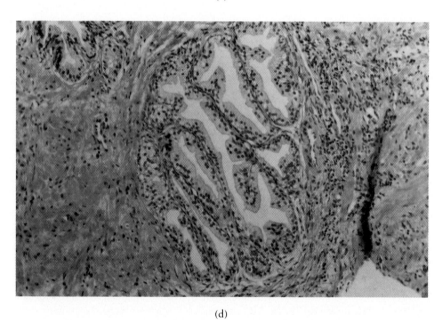

(d)

Fig. 9.5. C. ABC. Note loss of polarity and indistinct cell borders. Papanicolaou preparation. ×300. **D.** Histologic section. Note circumscribed collection of small glands with no intervening stroma. Hematoxylin and eosin preparation. ×125.

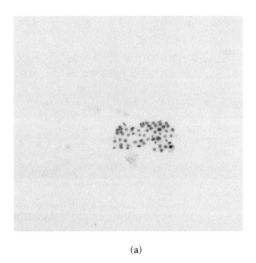

(a)

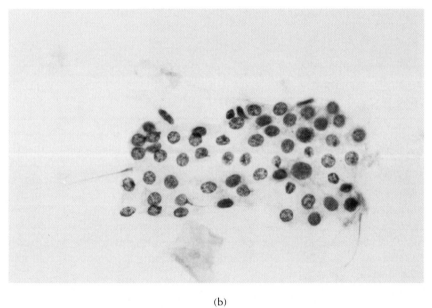

(b)

Fig. 9.6. Dysplasia. **A.** ABC. Note cell-poor specimen and cell cluster with loss of polarity. Papanicolaou preparation. × 125. **B.** ABC. Note cell cluster with anisonucleosis and indistinct cell borders. Papanicolaou preparation. × 300.

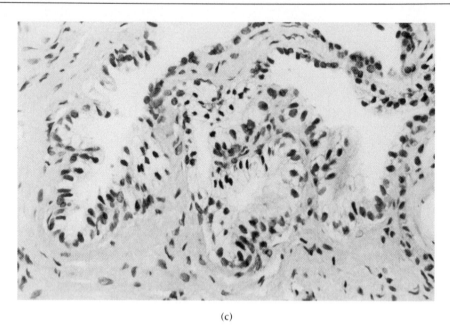

(c)

Fig. 9.6. C. Histologic section. Note glands lined by nonpolarized cells with irregular nuclei. Hematoxylin and eosin preparation. × 300.

INTERPRETATIVE TRAPS

False-negative diagnoses range from 5 to 30%,[36] whereas false-positive diagnoses are difficult to quantitate (see section on Histologic Confirmation of Prostatic Carcinoma, above). Problems in interpretation, not necessarily unique to the prostate, may arise for both the novice and the experienced investigator.[20] The most frequent source of error involves diagnosis of well-differentiated carcinoma (see Chapter 6). The dilemma of dysplasia will become an increasingly important issue as examinations of the prostate proliferate (see section on Dysplasia, above). Diagnostic problems also are attributable to technique, contamination, prostatitis, chemotherapy, and radiation.

Poor technique, occasioned by operator ineptitude or faulty specimen preparation, may result in false conclusions. Whoever obtains the specimen must be familiar with the procedure and the necessity for adequate and representative sampling by two or three biopsies. Cells distorted by poor fixation exhibit anisonucleosis, hyperchromasia, and nuclear membrane alteration. Diagnosis of carcinoma cannot be made on insufficient numbers of atypical cells or on poorly preserved cells.

Alteration of any phase of a standard procedure may produce an unanticipated pitfall. In our laboratory, we always had distributed the specimen evenly over the slide by gentle sweeping motion with a second slide or wooden applicator; recently, however, we dispersed it only focally with a coverslip (see Chapter 2, Fig. 2.4).

TABLE 9.1. Interpretative Traps

False-Negatives	False-Positives
Well-differentiated carcinoma	Faulty specimen fixation
Inadequate NAB technique	Altered technique
Carcinoma with prostatitis	Benign seminal vesicle or rectal cells
Radiation fibrosis	Prostatitis
	Radiation effect
	Chemotherapeutic effect

This modification led to enhanced cellularity which initially resulted in several erroneous suspicious reports (Fig. 9.7). Thus, technique constancy plays a role in accurate diagnosis.

Benign and malignant cells from sources outside the prostate may create diagnostic dilemmas. Contamination from the seminal vesicles introduces benign cells which mimic characteristics of prostatic carcinoma (see Chapter 3). The benign, large, isolated cells with irregular, hyperchromatic nuclei from seminal vesicles may cause an erroneous diagnosis,[9,21,22] but the pitfall is avoided by recognition of lipochrome granules in the cytoplasm and a sperm diathesis (Figs. 9.8 and 9.9). We suggest, however, that these contaminated aspirates be repeated; the biopsy needle may have been positioned incorrectly, or sparse malignant cells may be construed as pleomorphic cells of seminal vesicle origin.

Benign cells from the rectum may create an interpretative trap.[2] These cells with prominent nucleoli may congregate in small groups or form acini suggestive of well-differentiated prostatic carcinoma (Fig. 9.10). Observation of cellular elongation and characteristic palisade formation of similar cells usually prevents erroneous diagnosis (see Chapter 3). Rectal cells are negative to prostatic acid phosphatase by the immunoperoxidese technique (see Chapter 7). Alien malignant cells may also confuse diagnosis. The aspirating needle may puncture a carcinoma which invades the prostate or penetrate a carcinoma beyond its confines (see Chapter 6, section on Secondary Carcinomas).

Prostatitis induces a cellular pattern which may be difficult to differentiate from carcinoma (see Chapter 5). The cell-rich specimen is composed of cells, loosely cohesive because of edema, with anisonucleosis, prominent nucleoli, and most minor criteria of malignancy (see Chapter 6), although nuclear membranes usually are smooth. Accompanying histiocytes may be mistaken for malignant cells because of their isolation, pleomorphism, and prominent nucleoli. Epstein[11] erred in diagnosis of her first eight cases of prostatitis, and other authors[2,10] reported similar experiences. Thus, in the presence of many inflammatory cells, atypical cell groups should not be attributed to carcinoma unless they show all major criteria of malignancy. Conversely, isolated small cells from poorly differentiated carcinoma, surrounded by a few inflammatory cells, should not be mistaken for cells from prostatitis. When the diagnosis is equivocal, the patient should receive antibiotics and NAB should be repeated (Figs. 9.11–9.13).

Cellular alterations may be found after treatment with chemotherapeutic agents. Koss et al[24] described myleran-engendered pleomorphism with nuclear enlargement and hyperchromasia in exfoliated cells from the cervix, urinary tract, and lung. These changes, produced by an array of chemotherapeutic agents, also are observed in aspirates. The chemically altered cell often can be distinguished from the malignant cell by a glassy-appearing nucleus without distinct chromatin granules or a prominent nucleolus. After chemotherapy, however, most criteria of malignancy should be present before diagnosis of carcinoma.

Radiation may cause either a false-negative or a false-positive diagnosis. Postradiation fibromatosis may enmesh the carcinoma and result in a cell-poor ABC without malignant cells. On the other hand, radiation may produce bizarre but benign cells. Graham,[13] in a classic treatise describing irradiated cells exfoliated from the vaginal mucosa, found an initial increase in the quantity and extent of pleomorphic malignant cells and also many intra- and extracellular neutrophils, histiocytes, and multinucleated giant cells. In addition, there were benign cells with aberrant shapes, vacuolated cytoplasm, and vesicular nuclei with clumped chromatin. Although the malignant cells disappeared after 3 months of successful treatment, the atypical benign cells and inflammatory cells sometimes persisted for years. Similar changes are seen in ABC.[33] The prostatic aspirate from both the successfully treated and the recurrent carcinoma may be relatively scant. During the first 3–6 months, irradiated tumor cells may become bizarre and very large. Multiple or single nuclei with macronucleoli are irregular, and pleomorphic naked nuclei are frequent. Dyshesion usually suggests recurrence, and cells collect in small sheets or are isolated. Benign cells may have atypical features but lack well-preserved, eosinophilic nucleoli, the most significant sign of viable tumor cells. Apparent hyperchromasia or marked clumping of chromatin often is associated with degeneration. Zajicek[37] reported that pleomorphic naked nuclei were often seen after successful radiation treatment, but atypical cells with cytoplasm usually indicated recurrence. Needle aspiration biopsy should not be performed for at least 3 months subsequent to radiation. When the morphology is equivocal, NAB should be repeated at trimonthly intervals, until the ABC can be interpreted without difficulty. A cell-poor aspirate without abnormal cells from a clinically suspicious gland following radiation also must be repeated to assure representative sampling of the indurated mass (Table 9.1; Figs. 9.14–9.16).

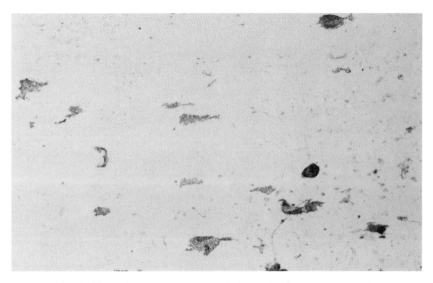

Fig. 9.7. Focal cell-dispersion preparatory technique, benign prostatic enlargement. Note cell-rich specimen composed of large, cohesive polarized sheets. Papanicolaou preparation. ×30.

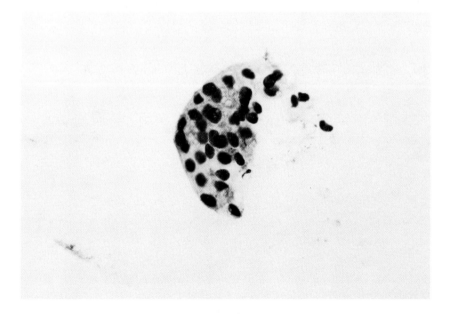

Fig. 9.8. Seminal vesicle cells, ABC. Note sheet with hyperchromatic nuclei showing anisonucleosis and irregularity but with cytoplasmic lipochrome. Papanicolaou preparation. ×500.

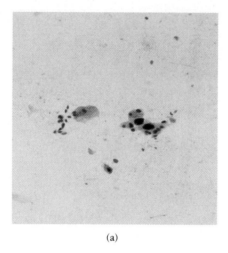

(a)

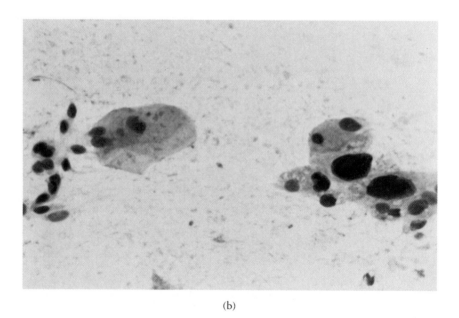

(b)

Fig. 9.9. Seminal vesicle contamination with well-differentiated carcinoma. **A.** ABC. Note seminal vesicle cells (right) and prostatic cells (left). Papanicolaou preparation. ×125. **B.** ABC. Higher-magnification view. Note bizarre nuclei of the seminal vesicle cells (right) and the loosely cohesive group of prostatic cells (left). Papanicolaou preparation. ×500.

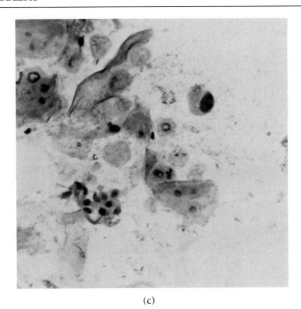

(c)

Fig. 9.9. C. ABC. Note group of prostatic cells with anisonucleosis and irregular nuclei (left) by contrast to the isolated large cell (center) from the seminal vesicles. Papanicolaou preparation. × 300.

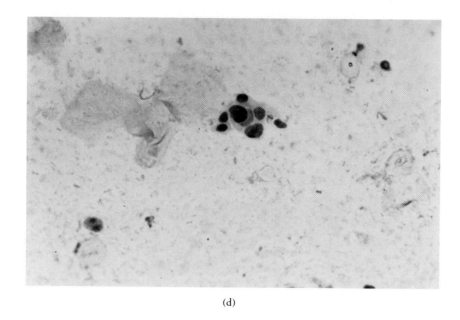

(d)

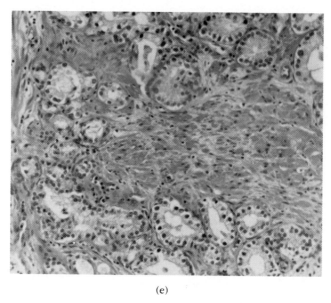

(e)

Fig. 9.9. D. Note central group of atypical cells, ?prostatic origin, ?seminal vesicle origin. Papanicolaou preparation. × 300. **E**. Histologic section, well-differentiated adenocarcinoma. Hematoxylin and eosin preparation. × 125.

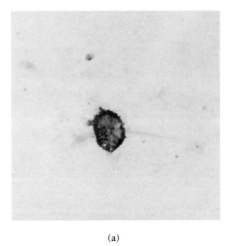

(a)

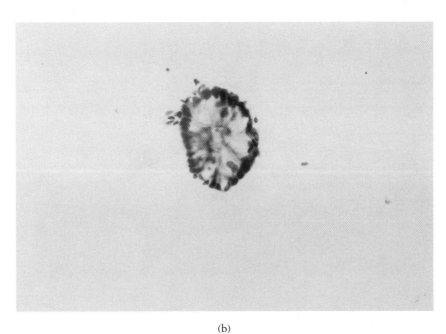

(b)

Fig. 9.10. Rectal contamination, ABC. **A.** Note small, regular acinus. Papanicolaou preparation. ×125. **B.** Higher-magnification view. Note elongated columnar cells with peripheral nuclei and cytoplasmic mucin. Papanicolaou preparation. ×300.

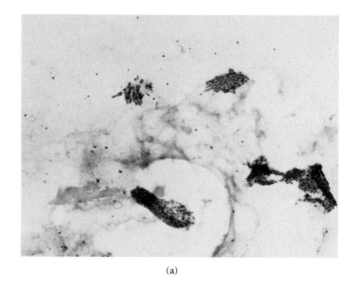

(a)

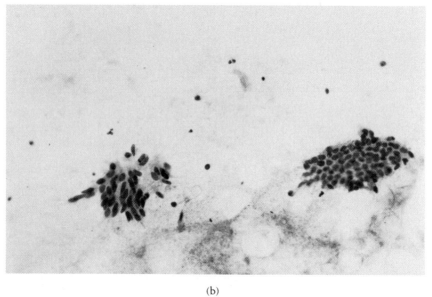

(b)

Fig. 9.11. Chronic prostatitis, ABC. **A.** Note relative cellularity with possibly dyshesive group (upper left). Papanicolaou preparation. ×125. **B.** Higher-magnification view. Note elongated palisaded cells (left) characteristic of rectal mucosal cells. Papanicolaou preparation. ×300.

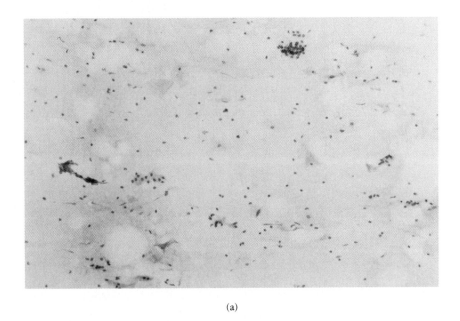

(a)

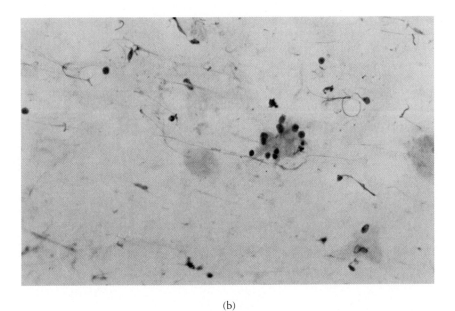

(b)

Fig. 9.12. Prostatitis with well-differentiated carcinoma. **A**. ABC. Note cellularity, possibly due to inflammatory diathesis. Papanicolaou preparation. ×125. **B**. ABC. Note microacinus within inflammatory diathesis. Papanicolaou preparation. ×300.

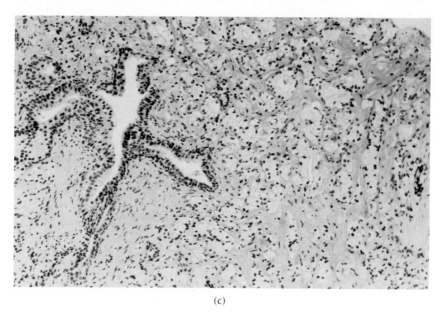

(c)

Fig. 9.12. C. Histologic section. Hematoxylin and eosin preparation. ×125.

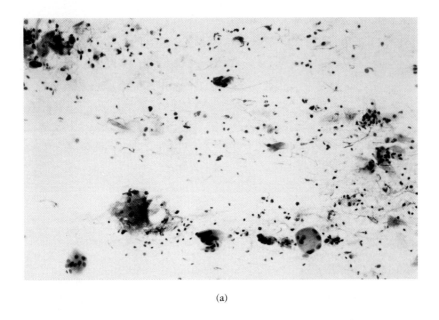

(a)

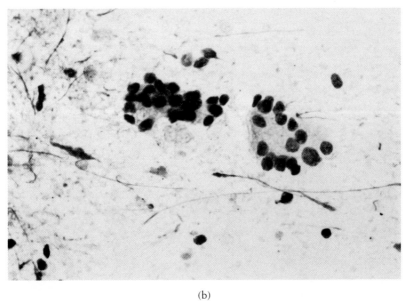

(b)

Fig. 9.13. Prostatitis with well-differentiated carcinoma, ABC. **A.** Note cellular aspirate with inflammation and prominent multinucleated giant cells (lower right). Papanicolaou preparation. ×125. **B.** Note microacinus. Papanicolaou preparation. ×500.

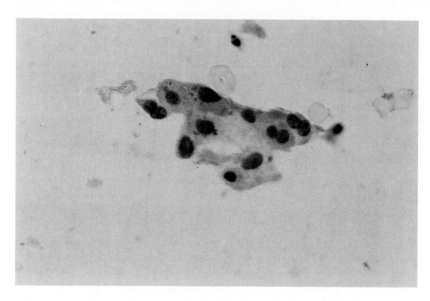

Fig. 9.14. Recurrent carcinoma following irradiation, ABC. Note cells with small secretory granules; benign or malignant? Papanicolaou preparation. ×500.

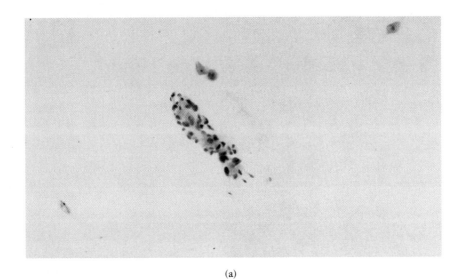

(a)

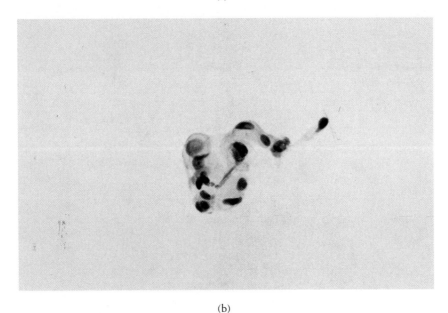

(b)

Fig. 9.15. NAB 6 months postirradiation, moderately differentiated carcinoma; ABC diagnosis: suggestive of recurrence, repeat 3 months. **A**. Note cell-poor specimen with cluster of atypical cells. Papanicolaou preparation. ×125. **B**. Note dyshesive cluster with pleomorphic nuclei. Papanicolaou preparation. ×300.

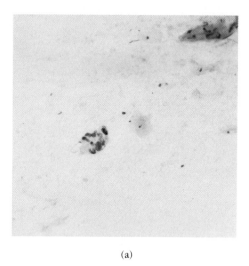

(a)

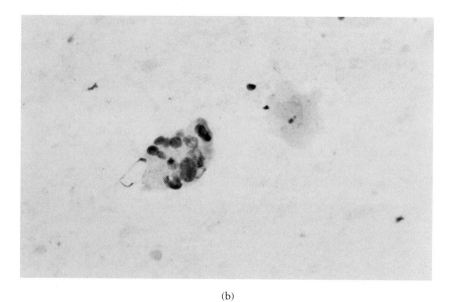

(b)

Fig. 9.16. NAB from patient with poorly differentiated carcinoma, 1 year postirradiation; recurrent carcinoma, moderately to poorly differentiated. **A.** ABC. Note sparse cellularity with single cluster composed of pleomorphic cells. Papanicolaou preparation. × 125. **B.** ABC. Note pleomorphic multinucleated giant cell with macronucleoli. Papanicolaou preparation. × 500.

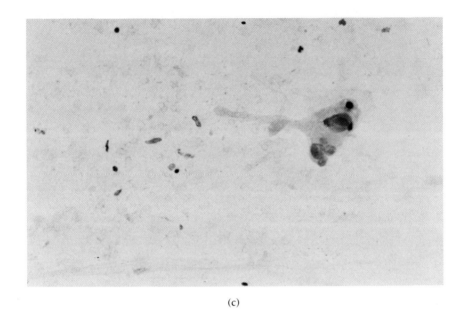

(c)

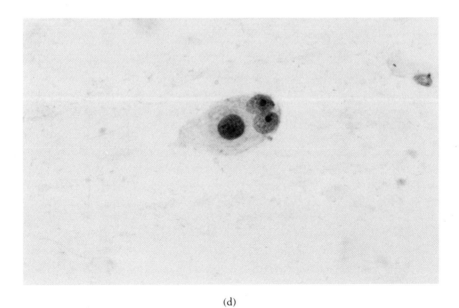

(d)

Fig. 9.16. C., D. ABC. Note pleomorphic multinucleated giant cells with macronucleoli. Papanicolaou preparations. ×500.

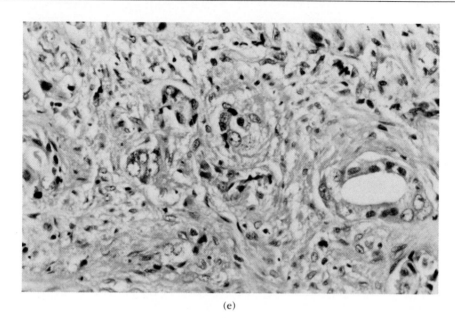

(e)

Fig. 9.16. E. Histologic section, original prostatic biopsy. Hematoxylin and eosin preparation. ×300.

REFERENCES

1. Ackermann R, Müller HA: Retrospective analysis of 645 simultaneous perineal punch biopsies and transrectal aspiration biopsies for diagnosis of prostatic carcinoma. *Eur Urol* 3:29–34, 1977.

2. Alfthan O, Klintrup HE, Koivuniemi A, Taskinen E: Cytological aspiration biopsy and Vim-Silverman biopsy in the diagnosis of prostatic carcinoma. *Ann Chir Gynaecol Fenn* 59:226–229, 1970.

3. Andersson L, Jönsson G, Brunk U: Puncture biopsy of the prostate in the diagnosis of prostatic cancer. *Scand J Urol Nephrol* 1:227–234, 1967.

4. Attah EB: Atypical stromal hyperplasia of the prostate gland. *Am J Clin Pathol* 67:324–327, 1977.

5. Brawn PN: Adenosis of the prostate: a dysplastic lesion that can be confused with prostate adenocarcinoma. *Cancer* 49:826–833, 1982.

6. Brawn PN: *Interpretation of Prostate Biopsies.* New York, Raven Press, 1983.

7. Cleary KR, Choi HY, Ayala AG: Basal cell hyperplasia of the prostate. *Am J Clin Pathol* 80:850–854, 1983.

8. DeGaetani CF, Trentini GP: Atypical hyperplasia of the prostate; a pitfall in the cytological diagnosis of carcinoma. *Acta Cytol* 22:483–486, 1978.

9. Droese M, Voeth C: Cytologic features of seminal vesicle epithelium in aspiration biopsy smears of the prostate. *Acta Cytol* 20:120–125, 1976.

10. Ekman H, Hedberg K, Persson PS: Cytological versus histological examination of needle biopsy specimens in the diagnosis of prostatic cancer. *Br J Urol* 39:544–548, 1967.

11. Epstein NA: Prostatic biopsy; a morphologic correlation of aspiration cytology with needle biopsy histology. *Cancer* 38:2078–2087, 1976.

12. Faul P, Schmiedt E: Cytologic aspects of diseases of the prostate. *Int Urol Nephrol* 5:297–310, 1973.

13. Graham RM: The effect of radiation on vaginal cells in cervical carcinoma. I. Description of cellular changes. *Surg Gynecol Obstet* 84:153–165, 1947.

14. Harbitz TB, Haugen OA: Histology of the prostate in elderly men; a study in an autopsy series. *Acta Pathol Microbiol Scand* 80:756–768, 1972.

15. Helpap B: The biological significance of atypical hyperplasia of the prostate. *Virchows Arch* [*Pathol Anat Histol*] 387:307–317, 1980.

16. Hoskins JH, Mellinger GT: Needle biopsy of the prostate. *G P* 34:88–92, 1966.

17. Karpas CM, Moumgis B: Primary transitional cell carcinoma of the prostate gland: possible pathogenesis and relationship to reserve cell hyperplasia of prostatic periurethral ducts. *J Urol* 101:201–205, 1969.

18. Kastendieck H, Altenähr E, Hüsselmann H, Bressel M: Carcinoma and dysplastic lesions of the prostate; a histomorphological analysis of 50 total prostatectomies by step-section technique. *Z Krebsforsch* 88:33–54, 1976.

19. Kelami A, Kirstaedter HJ: Erste Erfahrungen mit der Franzén-Nadel in der Diagnose des Prostatakarzinoms. *Urol Int* 24:560–568, 1969.

20. Kline TS: *Handbook of Fine Needle Aspiration Biopsy Cytology.* St. Louis, CV Mosby, 1981.

21. Kline TS, Kohler FP, Kelsey DM: Aspiration biopsy cytology (ABC); its use in diagnosis of lesions of the prostate gland. *Arch Pathol Lab Med* 106:136–139, 1982.

22. Koivuniemi A, Tyrkkö J: Seminal vesicle epithelium in fine-needle aspiration biopsies of the prostate as a pitfall in the cytologic diagnosis of carcinoma. *Acta Cytol* 20:116–119, 1976.

23. Koss LG: Book review commentary. *Hum Pathol* 15:398–399, 1984.

24. Koss LG, Melamed MR, Mayer K: The effect of busulfan on human epithelia. *Am J Clin Pathol* 44:385–397, 1965.

25. Lewis LG: Precancerous lesions of the prostate. *Surg Clin N Am* 30:1777–1782, 1950.

26. Lin BPC, Davies WEL, Harmata PA: Prostatic aspiration cytology. *Pathology* 11:607–614, 1979.

27. McNeal JE: Morphogenesis of prostatic carcinoma. *Cancer* 18:1659–1666, 1965.

28. McNeal JE: Origin and development of carcinoma in the prostate. *Cancer* 23:24–34, 1969.

29. McNeal JE, Kindrachuk R, Stamey TA, Bostwick DG: Premalignant lesions of the prostate (abstr). *Lab Invest* 50:39, 1984.

30. Miller A, Seljelid R: Cellular atypia in the prostate. *Scand J Urol Nephrol* 5:17–21, 1971.

31. Nienhaus H: Aspiration biopsy cytology of prostate carcinoma. *Cancer Res* 60:53–60, 1977.

32. Ortega LG, Whitmore WF Jr, Murphy AI: In situ carcinoma of the prostate with intraepithelial extension into the urethra and bladder; a Paget's disease of the urethra and bladder. *Cancer* 6:898–923, 1953.

33. Staehler W, Ziegler H, Völter D, Schubert GE: *Color Atlas of Cytodiagnosis of the Prostate.* Stuttgart, FK Schattauer Verlag, 1975.

34. Ullmann AS, Ross OA: Hyperplasia, atypism and carcinoma in situ in prostatic and periurethral glands. *Am J Clin Pathol* 47:497–504, 1967.

35. Ward JP: Franzén-needle transrectal prostatic biopsy. *Lancet* 2:327–328, 1973.

36. Willems JS, Löwhagen T: Transrectal fine-needle aspiration biopsy for cytologic diagnosis and grading of prostatic carcinoma. *The Prostate* 2:381–395, 1981.

37. Zajicek J: *Aspiration Biopsy Cytology. Part II. Cytology of Infradiaphragmatic Organs.* Basel, Karger, 1979, pp 129–166.

Index

Page numbers in italics refer to illustrations.